S0-BYF-694

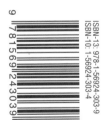

ISBN-13: 978-1-56924-303-9
ISBN-10: 1-56924-303-4

9 781569 243039

5 0 6 9 5

The NEW GLUCOSE

Revolution

Low GI Guide to
Sugar & Energy

**The Authoritative Guide to the
Sugar–Glycemic Index Connection—
and How to Use It to Your Advantage**

Dr. Jennie Brand-Miller

THE WORLD'S FOREMOST AUTHORITY ON THE GLYCEMIC INDEX

Kaye Foster-Powell

carbohydrates in Westernized diets portends a future acceleration of these trends. *The Glucose Revolution* challenges traditional doctrines about optimal nutrition and the role of carbohydrates in health and disease. Brand-Miller and colleagues are to be congratulated for an eminently lucid and important book that explains the science behind the glycemic index and provides tools and strategies for modifying diet to incorporate this knowledge. I strongly recommend the book to both health professionals and the general public who could use this state-of-the-art information to improve health and well-being."

—JOANN E. MANSON, M.D., DR.P.H., professor of medicine,
Harvard Medical School and codirector of Women's Health,
Division of Preventive Medicine, Brigham and Women's Hospital

∎

"Here is at last a book explaining the importance of taking into consideration the glycemic index values of foods for overall health, athletic performance, and in reducing the risk of heart disease and diabetes. The book clearly explains that there are different kinds of carbohydrates that work in different ways and why a universal recommendation to 'increase the carbohydrate content of your diet' is plainly simple and scientifically inaccurate. Everyone should put the glycemic index approach into practice."

—ARTEMIS P. SIMOPOULOS, M.D., senior author of
The Omega Diet and *The Healing Diet* and president,
The Center for Genetics, Nutrition and Health,
Washington, D.C., on *The Glucose Revolution*

∎

"*The Glucose Revolution* is nutrition science for the twenty-first century. Clearly written, it gives the scientific rationale for why all carbohydrates are not created equal. It is a practical guide for both professionals and patients. The food suggestions and recipes are exciting and tasty."

—RICHARD N. PODELL, M.D., M.P.H., clinical professor,
Department of Family Medicine, UMDNJ-Robert Wood Johnson
Medical School, and coauthor of *The G-Index Diet: The Missing Link
That Makes Permanent Weight Loss Possible*

■

"The glycemic index is a useful tool which may have a broad spectrum of applications, from the maintenance of fuel supply during exercise to the control of blood glucose levels in diabetics. Low glycemic index foods may prove to have beneficial health effects for all of us in the long term. *The Glucose Revolution* is a user-friendly, easy-to-read overview of all that you need to know about the glycemic index. This book represents a balanced account of the importance of the glycemic index based on sound scientific evidence."

—JAMES HILL, PH.D., director, Center for Human Nutrition, University of Colorado Health Sciences Center

■

"*The New Glucose Revolution* summarizes much of the recent development of dietary glycemic index and load in a highly readable format. The authors are able researchers and respected leaders in the nutrition field. Much that is discussed in this book draws directly from their years of experimental and observational research. The focus on dietary intervention and prevention strategies in everyday eating is an especially laudable feature of this book. I recommend this book most highly as an indispensable source of good nutrition."

—SIMIN LIU, M.D., SC.D., assistant professor, Department of Epidemiology, Harvard School of Public Health

■

"As a coach of elite amateur and professional athletes, I know how critical the glycemic index is to sports performance. *The New Glucose Revolution* provides the serious athlete with the basic tools necessary for getting the training table right."

—JOE FRIEL, coach, author, consultant

Other NEW GLUCOSE REVOLUTION Titles

The **NEW**
GLUCOSE
Revolution

LOW GI GUIDE TO

SUGAR AND ENERGY

The Authoritative Guide to the Sugar-Glycemic Index Connection— and How to Use It to Your Advantage

Dr. Jennie Brand-Miller
Kaye Foster-Powell

Marlowe & Company
New York

THE NEW GLUCOSE REVOLUTION LOW GI GUIDE TO SUGAR AND ENERGY:
*The Authoritative Guide to the Sugar-Glycemic Index Connection—
and How to Use It to Your Advantage*

Copyright © 1999, 2003, 2004, 2006 by Jennie Brand-Miller and Kaye Foster-Powell

Published by
Marlowe & Company
An Imprint of Avalon Publishing Group, Incorporated
245 West 17th Street • 11th floor
New York, NY 10011

This edition was previously published in somewhat different form in Australia in 2004
by Hodder Australia, an imprint of Hachette Livre Australia Pty Ltd.
This edition is published by arrangement with Hachette Livre Australia Pty Ltd.

The GI logo is a trademark of the University of Sydney in Australia
and other countries. A food product carrying this logo is nutritious and
has been tested for its GI by an accredited laboratory

The information in this book is intended to help readers make informed decisions
about their health and the health of their loved ones. It is not intended to be a
substitute for treatment by or the advice and care of a professional health care provider.
While the authors and publisher have endeavored to ensure that the information
presented is accurate and up to date, they shall not be held responsible for
loss or damage of any nature suffered as a result of reliance on any of
this book's contents or any errors or omissions herein.

The Library of Congress has cataloged the previous edition as follows:
Brand Miller, Jennie, 1952–
The new glucose revolution pocket guide to sugar & energy /
Jennie Brand-Miller, Kaye Foster-Powell.
p. cm.
Published in Australia in 2003 under the title:
The new glucose revolution sugar.
ISBN 1-56924-465-0
1. Sugar—Health aspects. 2. Glycemic index. 3. Blood sugar.
4. Energy metabolism. I. Foster-Powell, Kaye. II. Brand Miller, Jennie, 1952–
New glucose revolution sugar. III. Title.

QP702.S8B73 2004
613.2'83—dc22

2004042630

ISBN: 1-56924-303-4
ISBN-13: 978-1-56924-303-9

9 8 7 6 5 4 3 2

Designed by Pauline Neuwirth, Neuwirth & Associates, Inc.
Printed in Canada

CONTENTS

PREFACE

THE NEW GLUCOSE Revolution is the definitive, all-in-one guide to the glycemic index. This pocket guide shows you how the glycemic index (GI) relates to sugar and its effects on the body. As we explain in *The New Glucose Revolution*, the glycemic index:

- is a proven guide to the true physiological effects of foods—specifically carbohydrates—have on blood sugar levels;
- provides an easy and effective way to eat a delicious, healthy diet and control fluctuations in blood sugar.

This book offers more in-depth information about sugar than we had room to include in *The New Glucose Revolution*. Useful tips information appear here that are not in *The New Glucose Revolution*, including sample menus and the questions people most frequently ask about sugar.

This book is intended to be read alongside *The New Glucose Revolution*. In the event you haven't already consulted that book, you'll find it provides essential information about the glycemic index and all its applications.

◀ 1 ▶
INTRODUCTION

*M*ANY PEOPLE TODAY are convinced that sugar is a real "no-no"—one of the evils of modern diets and responsible (virtually on its own) for a multitude of human diseases. Others are not quite so negative, but still regard sugar as one of those things people can easily do without—because it's simply not necessary and you benefit by avoiding it.

These messages have been preached by doctors, dentists, nutritionists and health authorities for decades, and some still hold fast to these opinions despite the scientific evidence we now have. Their negative views of sugar stem from studies in the 1960s and 1970s that associated sugar with "empty calories," rapid weight gain (in rats!) and dental cavities. Nutrition science and public health have progressed markedly since then, but unfortunately some of the mud still sticks.

For the past twenty years, sugar has been the subject of close scientific scrutiny worldwide and the evidence from hundreds of studies indicates that sugar is not the villain it was once thought to be. In the opinion of the world's leading nutrition authorities including the World Health Organization (WHO) and the Food and Agriculture Organization of the United Nations (FAO), reasonable intake of sugar-rich foods can provide for a palatable and nutritious diet.

If we look at the recent scientific evidence objectively, the findings suggest that avoiding sugar may do you more harm than good. There are undesirable aspects of diets that are low in sugars. The vast array of sugar-free and "no added sugar" foods on supermarket shelves has not solved the problem of overweight and obesity. In fact, it could be said that they have exacerbated the problem.

In this book we take a look at the scientifically proven breakthroughs about sugar and energy; dispel some common myths; reveal why it's high time to get rid of the guilt; and tell you what you really need to know about sugar, your health and blood sugar control, weight loss, dental cavities and behavior and mental performance.

Our intention is not to encourage an excessive amount of sugar. Excess of anything is not a good idea! We want to convince you that a reasonable quantity of sugar—about 10 percent of total calories per day—can be part of a well-balanced diet. Unfortunately, Americans eat more than that at present. Luckily, this book tells you how to make this lower amount a reality by offering sample menus for adults, children, and people with diabetes.

2
UNDERSTANDING THE GLYCEMIC INDEX

HOW THE GLYCEMIC INDEX CAME TO BE

The glycemic index concept was first developed in 1981 by a team of scientists led by Dr. David Jenkins, a professor of nutrition at the University of Toronto, Canada, to help determine which foods were best for people with diabetes. At that time, the diet for people with diabetes was based on a system of carbohydrate exchanges or portions, which was complicated and not very logical. The carbohydrate exchange system assumed that all starchy foods produce the same effect on blood sugar levels, even though some earlier studies had already proven this was not correct. Jenkins was one of the first researchers to question this assumption and to investigate how real foods behave in the bodies of real people.

The Pancreas Produces Insulin

THE PANCREAS IS a vital organ near the stomach, and its main job is to produce the hormone insulin. Carbohydrate stimulates the secretion of insulin more than any other component of food. The slow absorption of the carbohydrate in our food means that the pancreas doesn't have to work so hard and needs to produce less insulin. If the pancreas is overstimulated over a long period of time, it may become "exhausted" and type 2 diabetes can develop in genetically susceptible people. Even without diabetes, high insulin levels are undesirable because they increase the risk of heart disease.

Unfortunately, over time, we have begun to eat more "refined" foods and fewer "whole" foods. This new way of eating has brought with it higher blood sugar levels after a meal and higher insulin responses, as well. Though our bodies do need insulin for carbohydrate metabolism, high levels of the hormone have a profound effect on the development of many diseases. In fact, medical experts now believe that high insulin levels are one of the key factors responsible for heart disease and hypertension. Insulin influences the way we metabolize foods, determining whether we burn fat or carbohydrate to meet our energy needs and ultimately determining whether we store fat in our bodies.

Jenkins's approach attracted a great deal of attention because it was so logical and systematic. He and his colleagues had tested a large number of common foods, and some of their results were surprising. Ice cream, for example, despite its sugar content, had much less effect on blood sugar than some ordinary breads. Over the next 15 years medical researchers and scientists around the world, including the authors of this book, tested the effect of many foods on blood sugar levels and developed a new concept of classifying carbohydrates based on their glycemic index values.

WHAT IS THE GLYCEMIC INDEX?

The glycemic index of foods is simply a ranking of foods based on their immediate effect on blood sugar levels. To make a fair comparison, all foods are compared with a reference food such as pure glucose and are tested in equivalent carbohydrate amounts.

Originally, research into the glycemic index of foods was inspired by the desire to identify the best foods for people with diabetes. But scientists are now discovering that GI values have implications for everyone.

Today we know the glycemic index of hundreds of different food items—both generic and name-brand— that have been tested following a standardized testing method. The tables in chapter 17 on pages 103 to 118 give the glycemic index values of a range of common foods, including many tested at the University of Toronto and the University of Sydney.

THE GLYCEMIC INDEX MADE SIMPLE

Carbohydrate foods that break down quickly during digestion have the highest GI values. The blood-glucose, or sugar, response is fast and high. In other words the glucose in the bloodstream increases rapidly. Conversely, carbohydrates that break down slowly, releasing glucose gradually into the bloodstream, have low GI values. An analogy might be the popular fable of the tortoise and the hare. The hare, just like high-GI foods, speeds away full steam ahead but loses the race to the tortoise with his slow and steady pace. Similarly, slow and steady low-GI foods produce a smooth blood-sugar curve without wild fluctuations.

For most people most of the time, the foods with low glycemic index values have advantages over those with high GI values. Figure 1 shows the effect of slow and fast carbohydrate on blood sugar levels.

The substance that produces the greatest rise in blood sugar levels is pure glucose itself. All other foods have less effect when fed in equal amounts of carbohydrate. The glycemic index of pure glucose is set at 100, and every other food is ranked on a scale from 0 to 100 according to its actual effect on blood sugar levels.

The glycemic index value of a food cannot be predicted from its composition or the GI values of related foods. To test the glycemic index, you need real people and real foods. (We describe how the GI value of a food is measured below.) There is no easy, inexpensive substitute test. Scientists always follow standardized methods so that results from one group of people can be directly compared with those of another group.

In total, 8 to 10 people need to be tested, and the glycemic index value of the food is the average value of the group. We know this average figure is reproducible and that a different group of volunteers will produce a similar result. Results obtained in a group of people with diabetes are comparable to those without diabetes.

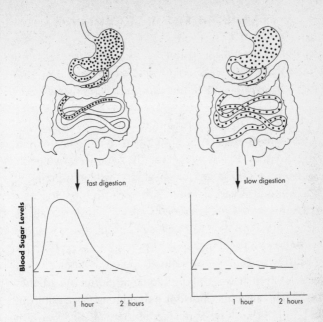

Figure 1. Slow and fast carbohydrate digestion and the consequent levels of sugar in the blood.

The most important point to note is that all foods are tested in equivalent carbohydrate amounts. For example, 100 grams of bread (about 3½ slices of sandwich bread) is tested because it contains 50 grams of carbohydrate. Likewise, 60 grams of jelly beans (containing 50 grams of carbohydrate) is compared with the reference food. We know how much carbohydrate is in a food by consulting food composition tables or the manufacturer's data, or measuring it ourselves in the laboratory.

The glycemic index is a clinically proven tool in its applications to diabetes, appetite control, and reducing the risk of heart disease.

MEASURING THE GLYCEMIC INDEX

Scientists use just six steps to determine the glycemic index value of a food. Simple as this may sound, it's actually quite a time-consuming process. Here's how it works.

1. An amount of food containing 50 grams of carbohydrate is given to a volunteer to eat. For example, to test boiled spaghetti, the volunteer would be given 200 grams of spaghetti, which supplies 50 grams of carbohydrate (we work this out from food composition tables or by measuring the available carbohydrate)—50 grams of carbohydrate is equivalent to 3 tablespoons of pure glucose powder.

2. Over the next two hours (or three hours if the volunteer has diabetes), we take a sample of their blood every 15 minutes during the first hour and thereafter every 30 minutes. The blood sugar level of these blood samples is measured in the laboratory and recorded.

3. The blood sugar level is plotted on a graph and the area under the curve is calculated using a computer program (Figure 2).

4. The volunteer's response to spaghetti (or whatever food is being tested) is compared with his or her blood sugar response to 50 grams of pure glucose (the reference food).

5. The reference food is tested on two or three separate occasions and an average value is calculated. This is done to reduce the effect of day-to-day variation in blood sugar responses.

6. The average GI value found in 8 to 10 people is the GI value of that food.

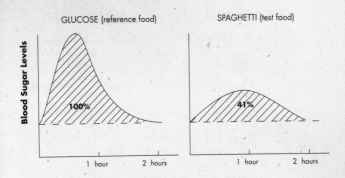

Figure 2. The effect of pure glucose (50 g) and spaghetti (50 g carbohydrate portion) on blood sugar levels.

■

A high GI value is 70 or more.
An intermediate GI value is 56 to 69 inclusive.
A low GI value is 55 or less.

■

Factors That Influence a Food's Glycemic Index Value

Factor	Mechanism	Food examples
Starch gelatinization	The less gelatinized (swollen) the starch, the slower the rate of digestion.	Low GI: Al dente pasta, brown rice High GI: Overcooked pasta, sticky rice
Physical entrapment	The fibrous coats around beans and seeds and plant cell walls act as physical barriers, slowing down access of digestive enzymes to the starch inside.	Low GI: Pumpernickel and grainy bread; legumes, and barley High GI: Bagels, cornflakes
High amylose to amylopectin ratio*	The more amylose a food contains, the less easily the starch is gelatinized and the slower its rate of digestion.	Low GI: Basmati rice, legumes High GI: Enriched wheat-flour products
Particle size	The smaller the particle size, the easier it is for water and enzymes to penetrate (the surface area is relatively greater).	Low GI: Stone-ground 100% whole-wheat breads and crackers High GI: Enriched wheat-flour products
Viscosity of fiber	Viscous, soluble fibers increase the viscosity of the intestinal contents and this slows down the interaction between the starch and the enzymes. Finely milled whole-wheat and rye flours have *fast* rates of digestion and absorption because the fiber is not very thick or sticky.	Low GI: Rolled oats, beans and lentils, apples, Metamucil High GI: Rice Krispies, kaiser roll

* Amylose and amylopectin are two different types of starch. Both are found in foods, but the ratio varies.

Factor	Mechanism	Food examples
Sugar	Sugar breaks down into 50% glucose and 50% fructose. Starch, such as enriched wheat flour, breaks down into 100% glucose. Therefore, the presence of some sugar in a food can lower its GI value. Sugar also inhibits the swelling of starch molecules, which also lowers its GI value.	Low GI: Sponge cake, pound cake High GI: Croissant, pancakes
Acidity	Acids in foods slow down stomach emptying, thereby slowing the rate at which the starch can be digested. Examples of commonly used acids are vinegar, lemon juice, lime juice, salad dressings, and brine (used in pickles).	Low GI: Sourdough breads, sourdough English muffins High GI: Enriched-wheat white breads, crackers
Fat	Fat slows down the rate of stomach emptying, thereby slowing the digestion of the starch.	Low GI: Chocolate or white cake from mix High GI: Angel food cake

3

WHAT *EXACTLY* IS SUGAR?

THE TERM "SUGAR" means different things to different people and the terminology can be confusing. In this book, as in everyday language, "sugar" refers to refined cane sugar, unless otherwise indicated. Sugar from sugar cane is a major source of this sweetener in American diets. "Sucrose" is the scientific name for the substance that contributes most of the sweetness in our diet.

The white granular powder extracted from sugar cane that we put in sugar bowls, cakes, cookies, and ice cream is similar to the principal sugar—and source of sweetness—in fruit, which contains a mixture of glucose, fructose, and sucrose. (The sugar in soft drinks comes from high-fructose corn syrup, which is a mixture of glucose and fructose. In the body, though, this mixture behaves exactly like sucrose.)

Sucrose is chemically classified as a carbohydrate and a simple sugar. Specifically, it's a disaccharide that's composed of glucose and fructose (see Figure 3).

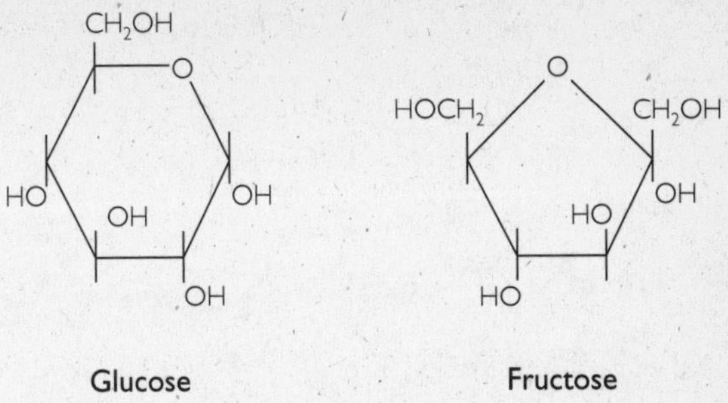

Glucose   Fructose

Figure 3: The chemical structures of glucose and fructose.

Types of Refined Sugar

- White (granulated)
- Brown
- Confectioners (powdered)
- Raw
- Molasses
- Pancake syrup
- High fructose corn syrup
- Turbinado
- Maltodextrins

The natural sweetness of fruit and honey comes from mixtures of sugar, glucose, and fructose. The mild sweetness of milk comes from another disaccharide, lactose, which is composed of glucose and galactose (Figure 4).

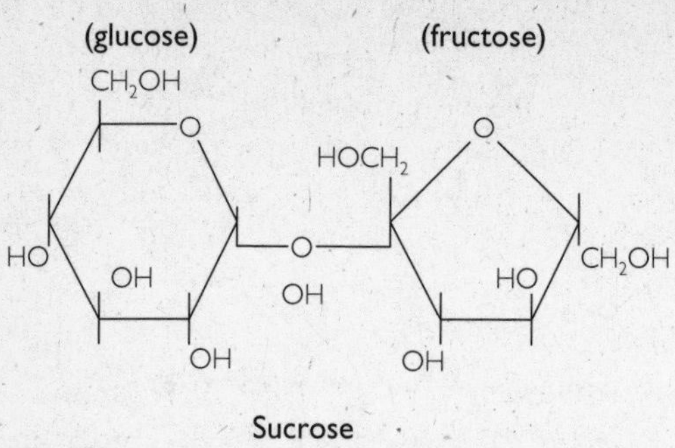

Sucrose

Figure 4: The chemical structure of sucrose (cane sugar).

Because sweetness comes from a mixture of sugars, not just sugar cane, we use many terms to define the original source:

▶ naturally-occurring sugars
▶ refined sugars
▶ added sugars
▶ concentrated sugars
▶ intrinsic and extrinsic sugars

If this confuses you, don't worry—it confuses the experts too!

HOW MUCH HONEY DID OUR ANCESTORS EAT?

It is possible that intakes of honey at various times during history may well have rivaled our current consumption of refined sugar.

In pre-industrial times, honey was the main source of

concentrated sweetness in the diets of many people. There are no precise figures for honey consumption because it was part of either a hunter-gatherer or subsistence economy, and of course, no records were kept then. Until recently, historians and food writers have proposed that it was a scarce commodity available only to a wealthy few.

However, a reappraisal of the archaeological evidence from the Stone Age to early modern times suggests that ordinary people ate much larger quantities of honey than previously thought.

- The ancient Egyptians made frequent use of honey in their spiced breads, cakes, and pastries, and for priming beer and wine.
- In Roman times, half of the recipes in a famous cookbook call for honey.
- In ancient Greece, those who died some distance from home were sometimes preserved in honey for transport.
- Medieval monasteries had so much honey that the excess was used to make vast quantities of a delectable drink called mead.

All of this suggests that there was plenty of honey around. During medieval times we know that honey was sold in bulk quantities such as gallons and even barrels—units unlikely to be used for a scarce commodity.

Even the poorest people could have had access to honey because bees often made their hives in hollow logs or broken pots. Wealthy landowners might own dozens of beautifully constructed beehives and employ a beekeeper (Figure 5).

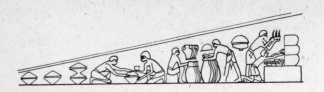

Figure 5: Ancient Egyptians made frequent use of honey.

Refined sugar may not have displaced more nutrient-rich items from our present-day diets but it may have displaced the only nutritionally comparable food—honey.

The Sugar-Fat Seesaw

DID YOU KNOW that fat and sugar tend to show a reciprocal or seesaw relationship in the diet? Research shows that diets high in fat are low in sugar, and diets low in fat are high in sugar. But studies over the past decade have found that diets high in sugar are no less nutritious than low-sugar diets. This is because restricting sugar is frequently followed by higher fat consumption, and most fatty foods are poor sources of nutrients.

In some cases, high-sugar diets have been found to have higher micronutrient contents. This is because sugar is often used to sweeten some very nutritious foods, such as yogurts, breakfast cereals, and milk.

A low-sugar (and high-fat) diet has more proven disadvantages than a high-sugar (and low-fat) diet.

ALL ABOUT ADDED SUGAR

Refined sugar is added to foods for more than just its sweetness. For example, sugar contributes to the bulk and texture of cakes and cookies and provides viscosity and "mouth feel" in beverages such as soft drinks and fruit juices. Sugar is also a powerful preservative and contributes to the long storage life of jams and confectionery.

In frozen products like ice cream, sugar has multiple functions: It acts as an emulsifier, preventing the separation of the water and fat phases; it lowers the freezing point, thereby making the product more liquid and "creamier" at the temperature at which it's eaten.

What's more, sugar retards the crystallization of the lactose in dairy foods and milk chocolate (tiny crystals of lactose feel like sand on the tongue).

In canned fruit, sugar syrups are used to prevent mushiness caused by the osmotic movement of sugar out of the fruit and into the surrounding fluid. Because sugar masks unpleasant flavors, sugar syrups are used as carriers for drugs and medicines, especially for young children who are unable to swallow tablet formulations.

In products such as yogurt and coffee, sugar masks the acidity or bitterness; it also balances the sugar-acid ratio in fruit juices and cordials.

Microorganisms also use sugar as the energy source for fermentation, so sugar is often deliberately added to foods for that purpose. It's added for the yeast in bread- and beer-making, but is totally converted to alcohol and other products in the process, so we don't end up consuming it as sugar.

What About Low-Calorie Products?

IT'S DIFFICULT TO produce low-calorie products because refined sugar is added to foods for so many reasons—not just for sweetness. So when manufacturers design a low-calorie, low-sugar product they find that many substances (e.g., preservatives, emulsifiers, antioxidants) need to be added to perform all the roles that sugar did alone.

LOW-FAT DIETS AND SUGAR INTAKE

One of the most important implications of the sugar-fat seesaw is that recommendations to reduce both sugar and fat may be counterproductive.

Most people are surprised to learn that the foods that provide most of our sugar intake (e.g. soft drinks, dairy products, breakfast cereals) are often low in fat. Similarly, the foods that provide most of our fat (e.g. meat, butter/margarine, fried foods) are often very low in sugar.

You may well be wondering how people in less affluent areas like Africa and China manage without sugar and still manage to eat a low-fat diet. While it's true that they eat a low-fat, low-sugar diet, their actual diet is far from balanced and optimal—their total energy and micronutrient intake is lower than it should be, often resulting in compromised growth and nutrition. High-starch diets are not a recipe for lifelong health and longevity.

Research shows that reducing your fat intake (especially that of saturated fat) is certainly more likely to result in desirable changes in body weight, blood lipids, insulin sensitivity and cardiovascular risk factors. But trying to reduce your sugar intake at the same time may not only compromise the effort to reduce fat, but reduce the palatability of your diet, and consequently the likelihood that you'll be able to stay on it over the long haul.

■

High-starch diets are not a recipe for lifelong health and longevity.

■

IS YOUR DIET TOO HIGH IN FAT?

Use this fat counter to tally up how much fat your diet contains. Do a tally for each day and then take an average. Using this fat counter, you will need to compare the serving size listed with your serving size and multiply the grams of fat up or down to match your serving size. For example, if you estimate you might consume 2 cups of regular milk in a day, this supplies you with 16 grams of fat.

FOOD	FAT CONTENT (GRAMS)	HOW MUCH DID YOU EAT?
Dairy Foods		
Milk (8 oz.) 1 cup		
whole	8	
2%	5	
non-fat	0	
Yogurt (8 oz.)		
whole milk	7	
non-fat	0	
Ice cream, 2 scoops (1 cup)		
regular	15	
low-fat	3	
fat-free	0	
Cheese		
American, block cheese, 1 oz. slice	9	
reduced-fat American cheese, 1 oz. slice	7	
low-fat slices (per slice)	3	
cottage, small curd, 2 tablespoons	3	
ricotta, whole milk, 2 tablespoons	2	
Cream, 1 tablespoon		
heavy	6	
light	5	
Sour cream, 1 tablespoon		
regular	3	
light	1	
Fats and Oils		
Butter, 1 teaspoon	4	
Oil, any type, 1 tablespoon (½ oz.)	14	
Cooking spray, per spray	0	
Mayonnaise, 1 tablespoon	11	
Salad dressing, 1 tablespoon	6	
Meat		
Beef		
steak, flank, lean only, 3½ oz.	10	
ground beef, extra-lean, 1 cup, 3½ oz., cooked, drained	16	
sausage, frankfurter, 2 oz., grilled	16	
top sirloin, lean only, 3½ oz.	8	

Lamb

rib chop, grilled, lean only, 3½ oz.	10
leg, roasted, lean only, 3½ oz.	7
loin chop, grilled, lean only, 3½ oz.	8

Pork

bacon, 3 strips, pan-fried	9
ham, 1 slice, leg, lean, 3½ oz.	5
steak, lean only, 3½ oz.	4
leg, roasted, lean only, 3½ oz.	9
loin chop, lean only, 3½ oz.	4

Chicken

breast, skinless, 3 oz.	4
drumstick, skinless, 2 oz.	3
thigh, skinless, 2 oz.	6
½ barbecue chicken (including skin)	30

Fish

grilled fish, 1 average fillet, 4 oz.	1
salmon, 3 oz.	3
fish sticks, frozen, 4, baked	14
fish fillets, 2, 6 oz, batter-dipped, frozen, oven-baked,	
regular	26
light	10

Snack Foods

Chocolate bar, Hershey, 1½ oz.	13
Potato chips, 1 oz. bag	10
Corn chips, 1 oz. bag	10
Peanuts, ½ cup (2½ oz.)	35
French fries, 25 pieces	20
Pizza, cheese, 2 slices, medium pizza	22
Pie, apple, snack size	15
Popcorn, fat and salt added, 3 cups	9

Total:

NOTE: The foods in this list have not been categorized as high or low GI since, with the exception of the snack foods, all other entries contain little or no carbohydrate, and thus are not ranked using the glycemic index.

How Did You Rate?

- **Less than 40 grams:** Excellent. 30 to 40 grams of fat per day is recommended for people trying to lose weight.
- **41 to 60 grams:** Good. A fat intake in this range is recommended for most adult men and women.
- **61 to 80 grams:** Acceptable if you are very active (doing hard physical work or athletic training). It is probably too much if you are trying to lose weight.
- **More than 80 grams:** You're probably eating too much fat, unless you're Superman or Superwoman!

4

IS OUR LIKING FOR SWEETNESS INSTINCTUAL?

SUGARS IN FRUIT and honey have provided carbohydrate energy in human diets for millions of
years—ever since primates began evolving on a steady
diet of fruit and berries in the rainforests of Africa 50
million years ago.

Our appreciation for the "sweet" sensation runs deep
in the human psyche. In literature and mythology,
sweetness is linked with pleasure and goodness, and in
everyday language we use terms associated with sweetness to describe the things we love (sweetie pie, honey-
moon). Our first food, breast milk, is sweet—in fact the
sweetest of all mammalian milks. Infants smile when
you offer them a sweet solution and cry if you give them
something sour or bitter.

Sweetness is not a learned taste: Everyone could be
said to be born with a sweet tooth. Scientists don't know
why we seem to prefer sweetness, but it may be related
to our brain's dependence on glucose as its sole source

of fuel. Perhaps those early human beings who were most able to detect sweetness were those most likely to survive. In fact, modern day monkeys that seek out fruit and berries have larger brains than those that survive on the leaves close at hand.

Our hunter-gatherer ancestors relished honey and other sources of concentrated sugars such as maple syrup, dried fruit and honey ants. Wild honey was so highly prized that they went to great lengths to obtain it.

Some Sources of Sugar in Early Human Diets

- Honey
- Parts of insects
- Honey ants
- Grape sugar
- Dates
- Maple syrup
- Sorghum
- Maize
- Sugar beets
- Sugar cane

As we mentioned earlier, our present use of refined sugars replaces our previous reliance on honey. In contrast, starches (the other form of carbohydrate energy) played a relatively minor role in human diets until we started cultivating staples such as wheat and corn some 5,000 to 10,000 years ago.

■

Sugars in fruit and honey provided the only carbohydrate energy in human diets for millions of years.

■

Sources of Starch

- Breads
- Breakfast cereals
- Cakes
- Cookies
- Grains (wheat, rye, corn, rice, and barley)
- Legumes (dried peas and beans)
- Peas
- Potatoes, potato chips
- Snack foods

THE ROLE OF SUGAR IN OUR DIET

Sugar plays a unique role in our diet. No other nutrient satisfies our natural (instinctual) desire for sweetness. There are also some healthy reasons to include a reasonable amount of sugar in your diet. It will help you:

▶ maintain an ideal weight
▶ reduce your intake of saturated fat
▶ maximize your micronutrient intake

Sugar also serves other roles in our food supply, too. It acts as a preservative, adds texture and improves the flavors of many foods. When we take the sugar out of foods we have to add other ingredients to do the job: We sometimes need intense sweeteners that help to replace the original sweetness; fat or maltodextrins to replace the bulk and texture; or preservatives to replace sugar's antimicrobial properties.

What Is a Reasonable Intake?

A REASONABLE INTAKE of sugar would come to no more than about 9 to 12 teaspoons of refined sugar a day. (Since we already eat too much sugar, it would be a good idea for most of us to stick to the lower end of that range.) That amount includes all sources of refined sugar—in soft drinks, candy, cakes, cookies, and frozen desserts, as well as what we add ourselves to tea, coffee, and breakfast cereals.

IS THERE SUCH A THING AS A SUGAR CRAVING?

The notion that we can become addicted to sugar and crave it constantly is based on the false assumption that sugar causes wild fluctuations in blood sugar—that it sends blood sugar levels soaring, floods the system with sugar and creates rebound or reactive "hypoglycemia" (low blood sugar levels). The low blood sugar is claimed to be responsible for the "craving."

This simply isn't true. Many studies show that

most sugary foods cause very moderate rises in blood sugar. Some types of bread and potatoes produce higher blood sugar levels than sugar. But no one ever hears about potato addiction!

If we crave sugar, it's because we humans have an instinctual liking for it—part of the hard wiring in our brains tells us that sweet foods are a safe form of energy. If we deny this instinct by deliberately restricting sweet food, it's not surprising that we find ourselves wanting it.

Studies of people who claimed to crave sugar actually found that the preferred foods were sweet-fat combinations such as cakes and cookies, which contain more energy as fat than they do as sugar.

Women appear to like these sweet-fat combinations more than men, who prefer meat and starch-fat combinations such as baked potatoes. This female preference may be related to a woman's greater requirement for carbohydrate during pregnancy and lactation. The fetus uses only glucose as a source of fuel (fat can't cross the placenta) and is entirely dependent on the mother for this glucose. During lactation, women secrete up to 70 grams of carbohydrate a day in the form of the sugar in milk.

So, if you think you have a sugar craving, you don't have to beat it or bust it. Enjoy everything in moderation!

■

If you have a sugar craving you don't have to beat it or bust it. Enjoy everything in moderation!

■

THE RISE OF REFINED SUGAR

Refined sugar is also known as table sugar, cane sugar or beet sugar. Sugar cane was one of the first foods that we began to cultivate deliberately (no prize for guessing why!). Sugar cane was first grown in Papua New Guinea 10,000 years ago, and the practice spread gradually to Egypt (2,300 years ago), Arabia (1,300 years ago) and Japan (1,100 years ago). Sugar beet, the main source of refined sugar in cool climates, was first cultivated in Europe 500 years ago.

Sugar cane and sugar beet have a naturally high content of sugar (about 16 percent) and have been commercially exploited as concentrated sources of sugar since 1600. Unfortunately, slaves harvested the crops, and were the main source of labor. Prior to this, refined sugar was a rare and expensive commodity and honey was much cheaper.

Sugar consumption increased dramatically in Europe beginning in the second half of the 18th century and replaced honey as the major source of sweetness. Our consumption levels peaked around 1900 and have remained, with minor variations, much the same for the past 100 years. Since 1970, though, corn syrup solids (glucose syrups made from hydrolyzed corn starch) and high-fructose corn syrup have partially replaced some of the refined sugar in manufactured products.

■

Soft drinks (10 to 12 percent sugar) are less
concentrated sources of sugar than either sugar cane
or sugar beet (16 percent sugar).

■

HOW MUCH SUGAR DO WE EAT?

According to the USDA's Human Nutrition Research
Center, Americans eat an average of 20 teaspoons of
added sugar a day—or about 16 percent of calories.

Unfortunately, this amount is higher than the amount
considered acceptable by health authorities all over the
world, including those in the United States. Public
health experts suggest that our intake should be no more
than 9 to 12 teaspoons of added sugar a day, or about 10
percent of total calories. (It's a good idea for most of us
to stick to the lower end of those ranges, since we
already tend to eat too much sugar.)

Use the menus on pages 44 to 48 to help bring your
sugar intake back in line with international guidelines.

◀ 5 ▶
THE IMPORTANCE
OF BLOOD SUGAR

A NORMAL BLOOD SUGAR (glucose) level is our life-
line. It allows our brains, red cells and other sys-
tems to function properly. If our blood sugar levels drop
too low, brain function is compromised and we suffer a
range of symptoms, including sweating and nausea. If it
continues to drop, coma and death result.

On the other hand, if blood sugar levels are too high
for too long, then our eyesight, kidneys, and heart function are affected. We get the glucose in our blood from
our diets and from the liver, where it's synthesized.

■ ■ ■

Blood Sugar or Blood Glucose?

BLOOD SUGAR AND blood glucose mean exactly the same thing. In this book we use the term blood sugar because it is the one most familiar to the public.

Consuming sugar (and any other carbohydrate that includes starch) produces hormonal responses that not only help the body take up this new source of energy and but also limit the rise in blood sugar levels.

Insulin plays an important role in bringing blood sugar levels back to normal after a meal by "opening the gates" and transporting glucose from the blood into the cells. Insulin also signals the liver to stop making glucose molecules and halts the breakdown of fat as a source of energy.

During the 3 to 4 hours after a meal, the amount of carbohydrate we consume (whether as starch or sugar) far exceeds the amount of carbohydrate that our cells are able to oxidize. As a result, much of the dietary carbohydrate-derived glucose is stored as glycogen in the liver and skeletal muscles and is subsequently released and oxidized within the next 12 hours.

That means that what happens to sugar in your body is the same as with all other dietary carbohydrates. The carbohydrates:

- oxidize (burn) in the tissues as a source of energy
- are stored as glycogen in liver and muscle cells
- get recycled in the liver for the synthesis of new glucose molecules (this is quite an active pathway)

▶ are converted and stored as fat mainly in the liver (under unusual circumstances only)

The body's glycogen reserves are small (usually one-half to one pound for a 110- to 154-pound adult; higher in trained athletes). The capacity to store more can be developed by exercise, training and diet.

A normal diet provides about 200 to 300 grams of carbohydrate a day. So within any 24-hour period, our bodies have totally oxidized the absorbed dietary carbohydrate, including sugar. Other body processes that help us dispose of dietary carbohydrate, such as conversion into fat or nonessential amino acids, are relatively unimportant in comparison.

THE FATE OF SUGAR IN YOUR BODY

The stomach empties the mix of foods and digestive enzymes into the small intestine where sugar is digested. The enzyme responsible for sugar digestion is called sucrase, which is located in the lining of the small intestine. The enzyme digests sucrose into glucose and fructose which are then absorbed into the bloodstream. Much of the sugar we add to foods has already been broken down prior to consumption; in fact, we actually swallow a mixture of glucose, fructose, and sucrose. Soft drinks are a good example.

The glucose molecule derived from sugar digestion is transported rapidly into the bloodstream while fructose is absorbed much more slowly. So slowly, in fact, that a large quantity of fructose (more than one ounce) by itself will cause diarrhea. The high fructose content of apple juice has been blamed for "toddler diarrhea."

Once absorbed into the bloodstream, glucose and fructose travel to the liver where some of the glucose and virtually all the fructose is removed. The body then burns the fructose as an immediate source of energy, while glucose passes into the circulation, entering the muscles and other tissues under the influence of the hormone insulin. In the muscle cells, glucose displaces fat as the source of energy and is burned to carbon dioxide and water. Under normal circumstances very little of the glucose is converted to fat.

BLOOD SUGAR RESPONSES AFTER A MEAL

After a meal containing sugar or starch, the blood sugar rises and reaches a peak within 15 to 30 minutes, then returns to baseline within 2 hours. In people with diabetes, this peak occurs later—between 45 and 60 minutes after the meal—because there is a relative deficiency of insulin. In the past, scientists assumed that refined sugar caused a more rapid rise in blood glucose levels than starchy foods or naturally occurring sources of sugars like fruit. Further research has proven this assumption incorrect.

Most starchy foods, including potatoes, bread and many breakfast cereals are digested and absorbed rapidly and the blood sugar response is almost as high as that seen with an equivalent amount of pure glucose. Foods containing refined sugar, such as soft drinks and ice cream, have been shown to give moderate rises in blood sugar, on average less than that of bread. (Remember, though: Americans in general need to eat less sugar. Let this book help you follow more reasonable guidelines.)

In addition, the blood sugar response to some foods containing refined sugars is similar to that of foods containing naturally occurring sugars (Figure 6).

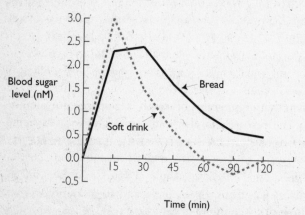

Figure 6: Comparison of blood sugar responses after 50 grams of carbohydrate in the form of sucrose or bread. (Notice the line for bread is higher from 20 to 120 minutes; this prolonged interval of increased blood sugar actually creates an excess of blood sugar over a extended period of time.)

In a study of more than 300 people with diabetes, the researchers found that a diet's GI value was linked to the percentage of carbohydrate consumed as sugars. The higher the sugars from all sources (both refined and naturally occurring), the lower the overall diet's GI value. This fact may be shocking, but it's because most common starchy foods, even whole grain versions, have high GI values.

Why? Well, consider that half of a sugar molecule is fructose and half is glucose. Fructose has very little effect on blood glucose levels. Starch, on the other hand, is made up of strings of glucose molecules. So gram for gram, sugar contains only half the glucose molecules of starch. When we consume 50 grams of starch as potatoes, we eat the equivalent of 50 grams of glucose (the starch is rapidly digested to glucose in the small intestine). When we eat 50 grams of sucrose, we eat the equivalent of only 25 grams of glucose, irrespective of the rate of digestion. So it's no surprise that the effect on blood glucose of 25 grams of glucose will be much lower than that of 50 grams of starch or glucose equivalents.

The researchers also found that glycosylated hemoglobin levels in the blood (the best measure of diabetes control) were found to be directly related to the diet's GI value. That is, those people eating the diets with the lowest GI values (those with higher sugar intake) had the best diabetes control.

This finding goes against many health professionals' recommendations concerning sugar and diabetes. Even the American Diabetes Association says that the amount of carbohydrate in a meal is more important than whether it's sugar or starch. Our message that you can allow yourself a moderate amount of sugar in your diet (9 to 12 teaspoons a day) is backed up by dozens of studies showing that sugar—in reasonable amounts—does not compromise diabetes control.

◀ 6 ▶
GLYCEMIC INDEX TABLES FOR SUGAR AND ENERGY

*A*S WE MENTIONED earlier, the glycemic index is used to classify foods according to their ability to raise the level of sugars in the blood, and we test all foods in equivalent carbohydrate portions according to standardized methodology. The following tables show the GI values of a range of common foods.

Foods Containing Refined Sugar	GI

Bakery Goods
Angel food cake	67
Apple muffin	44
Blueberry muffin	59
Banana bread	47

Cookies
Graham crackers	74
Milk Arrowroot	69
Oatmeal	66
Shortbread	64
Social Tea	55
Vanilla wafer	77

Breakfast Cereals
All-Bran	38
Cheerios	74
Cocoa Puffs	77
Corn Flakes	92
Crispix	87
Muesli, toasted	43
Muesli, non-toasted	56
Raisin Bran	61
Rice Krispies	82

Dairy Foods
Ice cream, 10% fat	61
Ice cream, low-fat	50
Milk, chocolate, 1% fat	34
Pudding	43
Yogurt, nonfat, fruit flavored, with sugar	33

Candy
Jelly beans	78

Foods Containing Refined Sugar	GI
Life Savers, peppermint	70
Mars Bar	68
Milk chocolate bar	49

Sports Drinks
Gatorade	89

Soft Drinks
Fanta	68
Coca Cola	53

Spreads
Nutella	33
Jams	51–55

Foods Containing Naturally Occurring Sugars	GI
Apple	38
Apple juice	40
Apricots, fresh	57
Apricots, dried	30
Banana	52
Cantaloupe	65
Cherries	22
Dates, dried	50
Grapefruit	25
Grapefruit juice, unsweetened	48
Grapes, green	46
Kiwi	53
Mango	51
Orange	42

Foods Containing Naturally Occurring Sugars	GI
Orange juice	53
Peach	42
Pear	38
Pineapple	66
Pineapple juice, unsweetened	46
Plums	39
Raisins	64
Watermelon	72

Starchy Foods with Little or No Sugars	GI

Breads

French baguette	95
Hamburger bun	61
Kaiser roll	73
Light rye	68
Pita bread, white	57
Pumpernickel, rye kernel	41
Rye bread	58
Sourdough rye	48
Stoneground wheat	54
White	70

Cereal Grains

Barley, pearled	25
Buckwheat groats (kasha)	54
Bulgur, cooked	48
Cornmeal, whole grain	68
Couscous, cooked	65

Starchy Foods with Little or No Sugars	GI
Corn, cooked	60
Taco shells	68

Rice

Basmati, white	58
Brown	50
Converted, Uncle Ben's	44
Instant, white	87
Long grain, white	61

Crackers

Kavli	71
Premium soda crackers	74
Rice cakes	78
Ryvita	69
Stoned Wheat Thins	67
Water cracker	78

Pasta

Capellini	45
Fettucine	32
Gnocchi	68
Linguine, thick	46
Linguine	52
Macaroni	47
Macaroni and cheese dinner	64
Ravioli, meat filled	39
Spaghetti, white	38
Spaghetti, whole wheat	32
Spirali, durum	43
Star Pastina	38
Tortellini, cheese	50
Vermicelli	35

Starchy Foods with Little or No Sugars	GI

Potatoes

Desirée, boiled	101
French fries	75
Instant potato	97
New, boiled	78
New, canned	65
Red-skinned, microwaved	79
Sebago, boiled	87
White-skinned, baked	85

Legumes and Beans

Soy beans, boiled	20
Lima beans, baby, frozen	32
Lentils, green and brown, boiled	30
Lentils, red, boiled	26
Black beans, boiled	30
Butter beans, boiled	31
Chickpeas, canned, drained	42
Chickpeas, boiled	28
Navy beans, boiled	38
Split peas, yellow, boiled	32

Snacks

Potato chips	54
Pretzels	83

Note: The complete GI Tables begin on page 100.

Label Reading 101

NOT SURE IF a food you're buying is high in sugar? Check the ingredient list on the label. If you see several of these words, or if any is listed as a first or second ingredient, you're probably buying a high-sugar product.

- corn sweetener
- dextrose
- fructose
- fruit juice concentrate
- glucose
- honey
- lactose
- maltose
- molasses
- sugar

7

EXPERT OPINIONS

*E*XPERTS FROM MANY countries have studied sugar's overall effect on health, including the United Nation's Food and Agriculture Organization (FAO) and the World Health Organization (WHO). A FAO/WHO group concluded that:

▸ Reasonable intake of sugar-rich foods can help to create a palatable and nutritious diet.

In addition, the American panel concluded that:

▸ At the levels normally consumed, sugar has no effect on disease risk, apart from dental cavities.

WHAT THESE RECOMMENDATIONS MEAN

That means you should consume no more than about 9 to 12 teaspoons of sugar per day from sources including soft drinks, breakfast cereals, and bakery products. As we discussed earlier, the average level of consumption in the U.S. is above this target, so stick closer to 9 to 12 teaspoons or less, if possible.

The difficulty is that the public and some health authorities remain concerned about the health effect of sugars, especially in relation to diabetes and dental disease.

DON'T GO OVERBOARD!

We don't mean to suggest that you should indulge in an excessive amount of sugar simply because sugar restriction is unnecessary. Far from it! But we do want to take the pressure off. Your normal instincts should guide you to eat a reasonable quantity of sugar—about 10 percent of calories a day.

To give you a guide to what this means in practice we have provided the following menu and a list of the refined sugar contents of a range of common foods.

A ONE-DAY MENU CONTAINING A REASONABLE QUANTITY OF SUGAR

Breakfast
 1½ cups All Bran with extra fiber and 1 teaspoon sugar

2 slices 100% stoneground whole wheat toast with
   margarine
Coffee with 1% milk and 1 teaspoon of sugar

Snack
3 Social Tea biscuits
Tea

Lunch
Ham and reduced-fat cheddar cheese sandwich on
   grain bread
An apple
8 ounces unsweetened orange juice

Snack
A pear
Water

Dinner
Steak with potato, peas, carrots, and corn
2 scoops low-fat ice cream
Water or unsweetened tea

Snack
No-sugar-added hot chocolate with ½ cup mini-
   marshmallows

This menu contains about 50 grams (about 12½ teaspoons) of added sugar, provides 1900 calories, and
meets the recommended proportions of nutrients, with
24 percent energy coming from fat (recommendation:
less than 30 percent) and 57 percent of energy coming

from carbohydrate (recommendation: more than 50 percent).

The total carbohydrate content is 285 grams made up of 123 grams starch plus 155 grams sugars (60 grams added, 95 grams naturally occurring).

A REASONABLE QUANTITY OF SUGAR IN A 10-YEAR-OLD CHILD'S DIET

Breakfast
    1 cup of Coco Pops with 1% milk
    ½ banana
    4 ounces unsweetened fruit juice

Lunch
    2 slices rye bread with 1 ounce ham with mustard, lettuce, and tomato
    1 small apple
    Water

Snack
    1 cup of homemade popcorn
    1 cup of reduced-fat milk

Dinner
    ½ cup spaghetti with meat sauce
    Carrot and celery sticks
    ½ cup vanilla pudding with 1/2 unsweetened sliced peach
    Water

This child's menu provides about 40 grams (10 tea-spoons) of refined sugars. It provides 1500 calories with 25 percent of energy from fat and 58 percent of energy from carbohydrate.

A LOW GI MENU FOR SOMEONE WITH DIABETES CONTAINING A REASONABLE QUANTITY OF SUGAR

Breakfast
  1 cup of rolled oats with 1% milk and 1 teaspoon of
    brown sugar
  A fresh orange
  Tea or coffee with 1% milk

Snack
  2 gingersnaps
  Tea or coffee with 1% milk

Lunch
  2 slices mixed-grain bread with 2 tablespoons
    natural peanut butter
  8 ounces nonfat fruit yogurt
  Water

Dinner
  Pan-fried fish with spinach, tomato, and onion served
    over a cup of long-grain white rice
  Green salad
  Tea or coffee with 1% milk

Snack
> ½ cup low-fat ice cream with unsweetened canned pears

This menu contains 40 grams (10 teaspoons) of added sugar. The total energy content is 1550 calories; 22 percent of energy is from fat, 55 percent from carbohydrate. The fat content is 38 grams. The total carbohydrate content is 220 grams, with 112 grams from starch and 108 grams from sugars (added plus naturally occurring).

Refined sugar content of various foods (grams)

1 rounded teaspoon of sugar	6
1 tablespoon of jam	8
1 tablespoon of honey	20
5 squares chocolate	20
1 chocolate bar (average)	35
12-ounce can of soft drink (average)	45
1 cup of sweetened fruit juice	5
1 ounce undiluted cordial	18
1 granola bar (average)	8
1 Lorna Doone shortbread cookie	3
1 cream-filled sandwich cookie	5
1 piece of chocolate cake	11
1 cinnamon and sugar doughnut	7
1 piece of plain cake	7

Sources of refined sugars

Soft drinks, cordials, and fruit juice drinks

Sweetened dairy products (ice cream, yogurt, flavored milk, pudding)

Milk flavorings (such as Nesquik)

Sweetened breakfast cereals

Flavored toppings

Jams, honey, pancake syrup, Nutella

Cakes, cookies, and bakery products

Candy and chocolate

Frozen desserts (such as Popsicles, Fudgesicles, and Italian ices)

Table sugars: white, raw, brown, cube

Sources of naturally occurring sugars

Sugar cane

Fruit of any sort

Honey

Dried fruit (dates, raisins)

Breast milk (lactose)

Cow's milk (lactose)

Vegetables (some are higher than others, such as carrots, red peppers, tomatoes, sweet corn, and beets)

Maple syrup

◀ 8 ▶
DOES SUGAR PROMOTE ILLNESS?

*O*LD MYTHS DIE hard: Sugar has been implicated in either the promotion or exacerbation of any number of illnesses for years. But according to the United Nations FAO/WHO Expert Consultation on Carbohydrates (1998), "there is no evidence of a direct involvement of sucrose, other sugars and starch in the etiology of lifestyle-related diseases." Still, the fiction persists. Below, we discuss a few conditions for which some people think sugar is to blame, and the science that finally clears sugar's name for good.

■

Research has shown that certain blood markers of diabetes control were directly related to the diet's glycemic index: Those people with higher sugar intake had the best diabetes control.

■

DIABETES

Diabetes associations worldwide have now recognized that there is no need to strictly avoid refined sugar. This change of heart resulted from the unarguable scientific evidence that blood sugar responses after eating sugary foods were no higher than those recorded after eating starchy staples such as bread.

In longer term studies of people with diabetes, those who were required to eat 12½ teaspoons of refined sugar a day in tea and coffee had no higher average blood sugars than those people given artificial sweeteners. Even extremely large amounts of sugar (75 teaspoons) didn't compromise blood sugar control. We definitely don't recommend this amount: It just proves a point.

There's no evidence to suggest that refined sugar causes worsening of glucose tolerance, insulin sensitivity or diabetes risk in humans. There are studies in rats that support this idea, but the amounts of sugar fed to the rats (equivalent to 100 or more cans of soft drink a day) are so much higher than a human would ever eat or want to eat that the findings are really irrelevant. When rats are fed sugar at the upper levels of human consumption, scientists have noted no adverse effects.

The important point is that avoiding sugar has consequences of its own that can be far more serious than any
potential effects of eating refined sugar. In other words,
restricting sugar may actually be counterproductive in
people with diabetes. This is because of the sugar-fat
seesaw (restricting sugar is frequently followed by higher fat consumption) and because starchy foods often
have a high glycemic index value.

Past studies of people with diabetes have clearly
shown that they eat less sugar but more saturated fat
than the general population. The consequence, of
course, is that they die of heart disease caused by hard-
ening of the arteries. Some of you may be thinking that
we should all try harder to restrict both sugar and fat, but
this means people would likely eat more starchy foods to
fill the gap.

The trouble is, some starchy foods have a more beneficial effect on blood sugars than others. If starchy foods
with a high glycemic index (such as some types of bread
and potatoes) fill the hole left by sugar, then it may do
more harm than good. Unlike sugar, high-GI starchy
foods have been associated with increased risk of diabetes and heart disease in the general population.

Two large studies from Harvard School of Public
Health involving 65,000 female nurses and 50,000 male
health professionals showed that high-GI, low-fiber diets
were associated with double the risk of type 2 diabetes.
What's more, in the Nurses' Study, heart attack risk was
doubled in those people who ate a high-GI diet. The
harmful consequences for people with diabetes are likely
to be greater still.

The Official Position

IN 1994, THE American Diabetes Association published a position statement declaring that the use of sucrose in a diabetes meal plan does not impair blood glucose control. They said that calories from sugar must be included as part of a diabetic's overall carbohydrate intake.

■

Unlike sugar, high-GI starchy foods have been associated with increasing the risk of diabetes and heart disease in the general population.

■

A WORD OF CAUTION

Some sugary foods may have moderate GI values, but because people often eat them in large portion sizes, they can add a hefty load of carbohydrate. Soft drinks, for example, have a GI value of 50 to 70, but an 8-ounce serving contains 25 to 35 grams of carbohydrate and a glycemic load of 20 or more, which is quite high. Consider both GI and GL values when choosing the best foods for blood glucose control. For more details on glycemic load, turn to Chapter 16 on page 95.

BLOOD CHOLESTEROL

Most readers will be aware that high blood cholesterol levels increase our risk of a heart attack. The dietary component most clearly associated with increasing cholesterol levels is saturated fat; reducing saturated fat is the most effective way to reduce the risk of heart attack.

Sugar, on the other hand, has never been found to increase cholesterol levels. When we reduce saturated fat, we tend to eat more carbohydrate to replace the missing calories. In some studies, this increase in carbohydrate intake—either from starches or sugars—has been found to cause a rise in blood triglyceride levels and a fall in the "good" form of cholesterol, or HDL. That's not good, since these factors can act independently of cholesterol levels to increase our risk of heart disease.

High levels of "bad" blood fats, such as triglycerides, and low levels of HDL are especially harmful for people with diabetes, who more often than not have a high risk of heart disease despite normal blood cholesterol levels. As a result, some experts suggest that the best course of action is to avoid both saturated fat and large amounts of carbohydrate and to eat monounsaturated fat instead.

The push for eating more monounsaturated fat is why experts and the media promote diets high in olive oil. Indeed, people in Mediterranean countries who do eat more unsaturated fat and less carbohydrate than other industrialized countries have a low risk of heart disease. But their diet and lifestyle differ in many other ways that may act in unison to reduce heart disease risk.

For example, people in Mediterranean countries eat more fruit and vegetables, more pasta and legumes, more salads and vinaigrette dressings. All of these foods have a low glycemic index, so blood sugar levels are low. Also, because of these low-GI foods, there's less of a tendency for the carbohydrate to increase triglycerides and reduce HDL levels. That said, it becomes more clear that olive oil alone is not responsible for the reduced risk of heart disease in Mediterranean countries.

Some nutrition experts are concerned that diets high in sugar might increase triglycerides more than other carbohydrates can. The basis of this worry? Studies that incorporate very large amounts of sugars (providing one-third or more of total calories) have found higher triglycerides and lower HDL than when starch was eaten.

Furthermore, some people appear to be more sensitive to the effects of dietary sugars on blood fats than others. We need to examine these variations more closely before we can be absolutely clear about the role of sugar. In the meantime, however, you can be reassured that diets that contain more typical amounts of sugar (around 9 to 12 teaspoons a day or 10 percent of calories), have no special effect on blood fats.

■

When we reduce saturated fat, we tend to eat more carbohydrate to replace the missing calories.

■

BEHAVIOR CHANGES

Some people believe that sugar causes ADD (attention deficit disorder, previously known as hyperactivity). That opinion is based on two theories:

- a possible allergic response to sugar, or
- a low blood sugar "rebound" after sugar consumption

However, results from many published research papers that have studied hundreds of people do not provide any support whatsoever for the idea that refined sugar causes or exacerbates ADD or affects cognitive performance in children. It's interesting to note that even those children originally considered to be adversely affected by sugar showed no effects when the sugar was given to them in a double-blind situation. (In this case, "double-blind" means that no one—including the scientist, the child and the parent—knew whether the child was getting sugar or an inactive substitute.)

It's possible that a very small number of children may have distinct reactions and respond adversely to sugar. But any carbohydrate, including bread and potatoes, could also be to blame if it causes blood sugar fluctuations.

Not only does sugar have no effect on most children's behavior, there's even some evidence that sugar might actually have a calming effect, if it has any effect at all: Glucose or sugar seems to influence the distress associated with painful procedures in human infants. In one study, babies given a heel prick cried less and had lower heart rates when they were given a 50 percent sugar solution just before the procedure than babies given plain water.

■

There is some evidence that sugar may have a calming effect, if it has any effect at all.

■

MEMORY CHANGES

There is growing evidence that consuming glucose enhances learning and memory in both rats and humans. The effect is best demonstrated in elderly people and those with Alzheimer's, but is also seen in young adults, if the test is sufficiently difficult.

In one study, elderly people were asked to drink either a glucose- or saccharin-sweetened lemon drink and were then given a battery of neuropsychological tests that measured memory, overall intelligence, attention and motor functions. The glucose drink improved these folks' performance on both the logical and verbal memory part of the tests (there was no effect on attention).

In another study of university students, consuming glucose improved their recall of narrative prose by 40 percent.

SUGAR AND NUTRITIONAL DEFICIENCIES

Many people think that eating refined and other added sugars is a bad idea because they offer "empty calories"—that is, they provide energy but without vitamins and minerals.

It's logical to assume that sugar dilutes the vitamin and mineral content of the diet but the real question is whether it happens in practice. If that were true, then we would expect to find that diets containing the least sugar would have the greatest quantities of micronutrients. But many large well-designed scientific studies found that diets containing moderately large amounts of added sugars were the most nutritious: more so than diets either low or very high in sugar. Researchers found that the higher the sugar content of the diet, the higher the intake of some micronutrients, including vitamins C, B_2, and calcium.

One of the reasons for this paradox is that sweetened foods can be excellent sources of micronutrients—breakfast cereals and dairy products such as flavored milk, yogurts and ice cream are good examples. People are more likely to eat them frequently and in larger quantities when they're sweetened. Many of us know children who refuse to drink plain milk but gobble down a strawberry milkshake or hot chocolate. A couple of tea-spoons of brown sugar on oatmeal or a tablespoon of jam on toast encourages a child to eat nutritious, but other-wise fairly bland, foods.

The second reason that reasonable sugar intake equates with greater intake of micronutrients is the sugar-fat seesaw: That is, low sugar diets in practice are usually higher in fat. Fats such as cooking oils, butter, and margarines are essentially empty calories, too. Of course, they do contain some vitamins, particularly the fat-soluble vitamins, but their very high calorie content means they tend to dilute rather than enrich the rest of the diet.

That isn't to say, of course, that all higher-sugar diets supply an adequate number of micronutrients. The fact is, most Americans eat too much added sugar already and too few servings of fruits and vegetables each day. So, though sugar is not a demon, we would do well to aim for at least five servings a day of fruits and vegeta-bles and try to cut down on the amount of sugar we add to our food.

■

Added fats, alcohol, modified starches,
and even pure proteins
are often sources of "empty calories."

■

9
SUGAR AND OBESITY

THERE IS A widespread belief that sugar is particularly associated with weight gain and obesity. This view stems largely from early studies in rats and mice that showed water sweetened with sugar led to rapid weight gain—not really surprising because water laced with any form of energy, whether it's amino acids, starch or fat would do the same thing, because all forms of food contain calories. Milk causes rapid weight gain, too! But the deed was done, and sugar's reputation for causing exceptional weight gain was accepted by the public and scientific community at large.

It's become clear that rats and humans are very different in respect to fat-making enzymes. Rodents are very efficient in converting carbohydrates (such as sugar or starch) into body fat, while humans have only limited quantities of the necessary enzymes and do it only under unusual circumstances.

HOW WE STORE FAT

We create human fat stores by channeling excess fat energy to fat storage, not by converting excess carbohydrate into fat. We know this because our fat stores have the very same fatty acid composition as our diet. If our diet is high in monounsaturated fat, then our fat stores will reflect this.

If we eat an excessive amount of carbohydrate energy, some of it will be stored as glycogen in our liver and muscles and all of it will eventually be burned (oxidized) as a fuel source.

If we overeat a very high carbohydrate diet (which is rather hard to do because it's often bulky and very filling), then it's the small amount of fat in the diet that will be channeled to fat storage.

Even an exceedingly large meal of pure glucose (500 grams, the equivalent of more than a gallon of soft drink in one hit) doesn't induce a net gain in fat. If overfeeding of glucose extends for several days, glycogen stores do become full (at about 1000 grams) and only at this point does sugar convert to fat. But this artificial situation is unlikely to occur outside the laboratory.

In everyday life, a high sugar intake causes an increase in feelings of fullness, so food intake is decreased.

FEELINGS OF FULLNESS

One of the most robust findings in recent nutrition science is that sugars result in much greater feelings of fullness compared to high-fat meals that contain the same number of calories.

In one study, students ate as much as they liked from a tasty smorgasbord of either high-sugar foods or high-fat foods on two separate occasions. They were "blind" to the nutrient content of the foods and the true purpose of the study. The investigators found that the students ate far fewer calories overall when they ate from the smorgasbord of high-sugar foods.

In another study, students were given either a high-sugar or a high-fat snack and one hour later were allowed to eat from an array of appetizing foods. They ate significantly less when the earlier snack was high in sugars.

Scientists now say that fat is very easy to "passively overconsume." Of course a high-fat meal can make you feel full, even sickeningly so. But the point is, you would have to eat an excessively large number of calories before you'd feel full. We all know that it's all too easy to keep munching on those "addictive" high-fat foods such as chips and peanuts.

But we tend not to do the same thing with high-sugar foods—eating jelly beans and other sugar confectionery is much more self-limiting—many of us feel a little nauseous if we indulge to excess.

THE FINAL TEST

The final test of the theory that "sugar makes you fat" is to look at the association between sugar intake and body weight in the general population. It's important that we exclude the dieters from such studies because they will tend to muddle the interpretation of the findings, having altered their diet in an effort to lose weight.

Another study published in 2000 compared three diets:

a low-fat diet that was high in starch; a low-fat diet that was high in sugars (30 percent of total calories); and a control diet typical of usual intake. Nearly 400 overweight adults were followed for 6 months. At the end of the study, the control group had gained a little weight (about 1½ pounds) but both the high-sugar and high-starch groups had lost about 2 to 4½ pounds. There were also no differences in blood triglycerides or cholesterol between the diet groups.

A well-designed study involving over 10,000 Scottish adults showed that diets low in sugars were associated with higher body mass index (a measure of overweight). In contrast, the diets high in sugars were associated with lower body weight. In fact, there was a consistent stepwise relationship between the two factors—the higher the sugar intake (as a percentage of calories or in grams per day), the lower the body mass index. This applied to both refined sugar and total sugars from all sources. This did not apply to starch—there was no difference in starch intake in lean and overweight people.

In an Australian study of identical twins, scientists found little evidence to associate any dietary factor with the degree of overweight. But, when the twins differed in weight by more than 9 pounds, the lighter twin tended to have a diet higher in sugar than the heavier twin.

One recent study published in the *Lancet*, however, suggests that sugar—from beverages—may be fattening after all. Researchers followed a large group of children for about three years. They found that the children who drank the most sugar-sweetened beverages (not total sugars) gained the most body fat over time. Although some experts were critical of the study design, some evidence does suggest that humans may be more susceptible to fat gain from sweetened liquids than from sweetened solids. If this is true, then all beverages containing sugar or other nutrients, including alcohol, milk, and fruit juices, may cause weight gain.

We can cite many other studies that show this inverse association between sugars and weight status. Of course, all of them are open to the criticism that conscious or unconscious "under-reporting" of sugar by the heaviest people is responsible for the trend. However, the same can be said of fat under-reporting and yet fat shows a direct relationship to body weight in the same studies.

There's ample reason to incriminate high fat diets with overweight (passive overconsumption being one!), but no good scientific evidence to point the finger at sugar.

◀ 10 ▶
SUGAR AND DENTAL HEALTH

$\mathcal{M}$UCH OF WHAT we know about the relationship of sugars to dental decay was gathered before the "fluoride era." Sugar's bad reputation seemed confirmed at that time when research showed a strong relationship between the number of decayed and missing teeth and the amount of sugar people ate.

In the post-fluoride era, it's clear that the best way to promote healthy teeth is to drink fluoridated water, floss daily, brush your teeth twice a day and use a fluoride toothpaste. Total sugar consumption has less to do with it than we once thought. Dentists now recognize that all fermentable carbohydrates (i.e., both sugars and starches), can promote dental decay. More important, it's not the total amount eaten, but the frequency of eating and consistency of the food that determine its cavity-causing potential.

All fermentable carbohydrates, including sugars and starches, are capable of causing dental cavities.

Naturally occurring sugars in breast milk, fruit and honey are no different from those in candies and other sweets, and whole grain cereals and flours are just as responsible. The starches in breakfast cereals and potatoes, when caught between the teeth, help to start dental cavities. That's why it makes no sense to suggest that we reduce our intake of sugar while simultaneously recommending higher starch intake.

Indeed, the first archaeological evidence of dental decay appeared 10,000 years ago when humans first adopted farming and starch became a common component of the diet (and long before refined sugar came along). Even in those days some people lost all of their teeth to dental decay.

MECHANISMS OF TOOTH DECAY

Every time we eat or drink, we subject our teeth to an unavoidable "acid wash," because the bacteria in plaque ferment any leftover carbohydrate that remains on teeth to acid.

Acid formation begins within minutes of eating and gradually dissolves the enamel of the tooth's surface, but teeth strengthened by fluoride have the best defense against this acid. For the following half hour after eating, the acids are gradually neutralized by saliva and the tooth surface returns to normal.

Dental experts have shown that our teeth can put up with about four to six of these "acid washes" a day and still stay in good shape. If you eat all your fermentable carbohydrates at breakfast, lunch, dinner, and snacks throughout the day, then your teeth should theoretically stay cavity-free.

However, sticky foods such as lollipops that remain on the teeth or stuck between them for long periods promote tooth decay because the acids are continually being formed by bacterial fermentation. Hard candies aren't the only culprit however—dried fruit and carbohydrates can stick between teeth too! (Foods like cornflakes can produce just as much acid as sugary foods.) Similarly, if we sip sweet drinks for hours (whether a soft drink or juice), we prolong the acid bath and increase the risk of cavities.

Some babies develop severe tooth decay by being continuously breastfed or bottle-fed throughout the night. If we eat very frequently, whether we're munching on non-sugary foods such as potato chips or naturally-occurring sugary foods such as fruit, we promote acid formation and dental decay. (In one study, dental decay was found to be significantly greater in citrus and other fruit pickers compared to the neighboring workers on vegetable farms!)

■

Regular tooth brushing and flossing play a more important role in the prevention of tooth decay in the post-fluoride era.

■

Candies promote dental decay because you're more likely to eat them between meals than any other type of food. Furthermore, many types of confectionery take a long time to dissolve in the mouth (hard candies), are sticky (such as jelly beans and licorice) or are sucked for long periods (lollipops). There's no doubt that frequent consumption of these foods will promote tooth decay even in fluoridated areas. The actual amount of sugar eaten may be quite small, but the effect is enormous.

If we decide to replace these between-meal snacks with more "natural" products such as dried fruit, or with starchy foods such as bread and crackers, we may be no better off: It all comes down to frequency of consumption between meals.

Public health strategies to reduce the incidence of dental cavities are far more likely to be successful if they emphasize using fluoride toothpaste and practicing good dental hygiene, rather than reducing our sugar consumption.

A WORD ABOUT LOW-CALORIE SOFT DRINKS

One of the most frequent ways people try to reduce their sugar intake is by drinking low-calorie soft drinks in place of regular varieties. If, by doing this, the intention is to reduce dental cavities, this isn't the way to do it. Low-calorie soft drinks are highly acidic, just like regular soft drinks and most fruits. The drink's acidic nature helps to dissolve the enamel on the tooth surface, even in the absence of bacteria and plaque. We've all heard the story of one famous brand of soft drink that completely dissolved a tooth overnight. Well, the same will happen with the regular or diet version of any soft drink.

The trend to carry and drink water (both free and expensive versions) instead of juice or a soft drink is a good idea: Many people, much of the time, walk around in a state of semi-dehydration that affects both mental and physical performance!

11

GOOD INTENTIONS

ONE OF THE main messages of this book is that well-meaning efforts to reduce our sugar intake may do more harm than good. Unfortunately, when we reduce our consumption of sugar—either consciously or unconsciously—we tend to increase our intake of high-GI foods (such as some types of bread and rice), or of foods high in saturated fat, such as cheese, crackers, and potato chips. Those foods may do more long-term harm to our health than sugar.

While many nutritionists feel that people ought to be able to reduce both their sugar and fat intake to low levels, only a small minority of the population actually does so in practice. Furthermore, this recommendation is based on the assumed superiority of starches to sugars—that high intake of starchy foods such as some types of cereals, bread, and potatoes always goes hand-in-hand with good health. Unfortunately, this isn't necessarily so populations all over the world that have high starch intakes are among those with the highest rates of protein-energy malnutrition and stunted growth. Furthermore, starchy foods with high GI values increase insulin demand and therefore promote the diseases of affluence—diabetes, heart disease and obesity. Sugary foods have lower GI values than most starchy foods.

■

You can use sugar to maximize your well-being and enjoyment of life.

■

THE RISE OF SUGAR SUBSTITUTES

Our emphasis on reducing sugar intake also fuels the demand for intense sweeteners to use as sugar substitutes. In China, the relatively new soft drink industry is based almost entirely on saccharin-sweetened drinks not only because sugar is more expensive in China but also because it is seen as something that should be avoided. While there's no evidence that intense sweeteners cause harm, there is actually little support for using them at all. We're still an overweight nation despite the number of low-calorie products that are on the market.

We spend millions of dollars on the research and development, safety testing and product development of foods incorporating intense sweeteners. In our opinion, this money would be better channeled into research on the real causes of obesity and diabetes and their treatment.

There may be a place for tooth-friendly candies made with sugar substitutes such as Isomalt, an artificial sweetener that's becoming more popular in the United States. Truth is, intense sweeteners are probably here to stay simply because nutrition and other health authorities continue to push the message that sugar is to be avoided if at all possible.

Our take-home message: Reasonable amounts of sugar (about 10 percent of total calories a day) need not be discouraged. That intake is associated with:

- the highest intake of micronutrients
- lower intakes of saturated fat
- a lower-GI diet
- a lower body weight (in some cases)
- "socially acceptable" food habits
- long-term dietary compliance

■

You don't need to beat it or bust it, and you can cut the guilt trip. The desire for sweetness in foods is a human one.

■

RID YOURSELF OF GUILT

It's okay to use sugar if it improves the taste of those very nutritious but rather bland foods—low-fat milk, yogurt, oatmeal, and other whole-grain breakfast cereals. Don't hesitate to put a tablespoon of jam on your bread, a little honey in your tea, or a sprinkle of sugar on unripe, sour or acidic fruit. And don't fret about the sugar in baked beans or canned fruit—these foods are good for you and if you are more likely to eat them because you like them sweetened, go ahead and enjoy.

It's a good nutritional rule of thumb to consider the nutrients your body will get from the nutrients you consume. Just don't forget your five servings of fruit and vegetables. If ice cream is your weak spot, choose low-fat, not low-sugar versions. If you want to "pig out" now and again, it's much better to do it on jelly beans and hard candies rather than on chocolate and potato chips.

12

THE BENEFITS OF LIVING
AN ACTIVE LIFE

A MULTITUDE OF changes in our living habits now means that in both work and recreation we are more sedentary than ever. Our physical activity levels are now so low that we take in more calories than we burn off, causing us to gain weight. Luckily, exercise is our ticket back to healthy living.

Regular physical activity can reduce our blood sugar levels, lower our risk of heart and blood vessel disease, lower high blood pressure, increase stamina, reduce stress, and help us relax. It's a good idea for all of us.

■

To lose weight you need to eat fewer calories and burn more calories—and that means getting regular exercise and leading a more active lifestyle.

■

THE BENEFITS OF EXERCISE

Most people could tell you at least one health benefit of exercise (reduces blood pressure, lowers the risk of heart disease, improves circulation, increases stamina, flexibility, and strength), but the most motivating aspect of exercise is feeling so good about yourself for doing it.

Exercise speeds up our metabolic rate. By increasing our caloric expenditure, exercise helps to balance our sometimes excessive caloric intake from food.

More movement makes our muscles better at using fat as a source of fuel. By improving the way insulin works, exercise increases the amount of fat we burn.

A low-GI diet has the same effect. Low-GI foods reduce the amount of insulin we need, which makes fat easier to burn and harder to store. Since it's body fat that you want to get rid of when you lose weight, exercise in combination with a low-GI diet makes a lot of sense!

HOW TO GET MOVING

Getting more exercise doesn't necessarily mean daily aerobics classes and jogging around the block (although this is great if you want to do it). What it does mean is moving more in everyday living. It's the day-to-day things we do—shopping, ironing, chasing kids, walking from the train station—where we spend the bulk of our energy.

Since so much of our lifestyle is designed now to reduce our physical exertion, it's become very important to catch bursts of physical activity wherever we can, to increase our energy output. It may mean using the stairs instead of the elevator, taking a 10-minute walk at lunch time, trotting on a treadmill while you watch the news or talk on the telephone, walking to the grocery store to get the Sunday paper, hiding the remote control, parking a half mile from work, or taking the dog for a walk each night. Whatever it means, do it. Even housework burns calories!

How Exercise Keeps Burning Calories, Even When You Are at Rest

THE EFFECT OF exercise doesn't stop when you do. People who exercise have higher metabolic rates, so their bodies continue to burn more calories every minute, even when they're asleep!

Besides increasing the incidental activity, you will also benefit from some planned aerobic activity, which causes you to breathe more heavily and makes your heart beat faster. Walking, cycling, swimming, and stair climbing are just a few examples. You'll need to accumulate a total of at least 30 minutes of this type of activity five to six days a week.

Remember that reduction in body weight takes time. Even after you've made changes in your exercise habits, your weight may not be any different on the scale. (This is particularly true for women, whose bodies tend to adapt to increased caloric expenditure.)

Whatever it takes for you to burn more calories, do it. Try to regard movement as an opportunity to improve your physical well-being—not as an inconvenience.

EXERCISE, DIABETES, AND
THE GLYCEMIC INDEX

We're talking about the everyday sort of moderate exercise that all of us should be doing. If you train physically hard a number of days a week and perhaps compete in sports you should read *The New Glucose Revolution Pocket Guide to Peak Performance*.

It is sometimes necessary with diabetes to eat extra carbohydrate when you exercise depending on the type of diabetes you have and the type and amount of medication you take. Often, you won't want to increase your food intake—because the exercise is intended to burn off some earlier overconsumption! (For people with type 1 diabetes, remember this will only work if you have enough insulin in your body and your blood sugars aren't too high to start with.)

You may need extra carbohydrate before you exercise, or, if the exercise is prolonged over an hour or more, you may need extra carbohydrate while you exercise, too. Whether or not you need to eat extra, and how much to take, depends on your blood sugar level before, during, and after the exercise, and how your body responds to the exercise—all of which you learn from experience. Discuss your situation and how best to manage it with a dietitian, diabetes educator or doctor.

If you need to eat immediately before exercise to bring your blood sugar up during exercise, it makes sense to eat some high-GI carbohydrate, such as a slice of regular bread, a couple of cookies, or a ripe banana.

If you plan to eat your last meal or snack one to two hours before your exercise, it makes sense to eat a low-GI meal to sustain you through the exercise, such as a sandwich made with low-GI bread, lowfat protein such as turkey breast or boiled ham, a container of yogurt, or an apple.

If you need to eat something quickly after or during exercise to restore your blood sugar level, use high-GI food—crispbread or rice cakes, a bowl of corn flakes or Rice Krispies, or a slice of watermelon, for example.

NOTE: Always remember to measure your blood sugar when you exercise to assess your body's response and judge your carbohydrate needs.

■

Exercise makes our muscles better at using fat as a source of fuel.

■

8 WAYS TO MAKE EXERCISE WORK FOR YOU

Your exercise routine will bring you lots of benefits if you can:

1. appreciate its benefits
2. enjoy doing it
3. feel good about your ability to exercise
4. make it a normal part of your day
5. keep it inexpensive
6. make it accessible
7. stay safe while doing it
8. do it with someone

◀ 13 ▶
YOUR QUESTIONS ANSWERED

Can people with diabetes eat as much sugar as they want?

Not as much as they want, necessarily, but perhaps more than you think. Research shows that moderate consumption of refined sugar (about 10 teaspoons) a day doesn't compromise blood sugar control. This means you can choose foods which contain refined sugar or even use small amounts of table sugar. Try to spread your sugar budget over a variety of nutrient rich foods that sugar makes more palatable. Remember, sugar is concealed in many foods—a can of soft drink contains about 40 grams of sugar.

Most foods containing sugar do not raise blood sugar levels any more than most starchy foods.

Sugar can be a source of enjoyment and help you limit your intake of high fat foods, but the blood sugar response to a food is hard to predict. Use the tables in this book and your own blood sugar monitoring as a guide.

Are naturally occurring sugars better than refined sugars?

Naturally occurring sugars are those found in foods such as fruit, vegetables, and milk. Refined sugars are concentrated sources of sugar such as table sugar, honey, or molasses.

The rate of digestion and absorption of naturally occurring sugars is no different, on average, from that of refined sugars. There is wide variation within both food groups, depending on the food. For example, the glycemic index of fruits ranges from 22 for cherries to 72 for watermelon. Similarly, among the foods containing refined sugars, some have low GI values, while others have high GI numbers. The glycemic index of sweetened yogurt is only 33, while each Life Savers candy has a glycemic index of 70 (the same as some breads).

Some nutritionists argue that naturally occurring sugars are better because they contain minerals and vitamins not found in refined sugar. However, recent studies which have analyzed high-sugar and low-sugar diets clearly show that the diets overall contain similar amounts of micronutrients. Studies have shown that people who eat moderate amounts of refined sugars have perfectly adequate micronutrient intakes.

I've always heard that sugar is fattening. Is it?

No. Sugar has no special fattening properties—in fact, it is no more likely to be turned into fat than any other carbohydrate. Sugar, which you'll often find in foods high in calories and fat, may sometimes seem to be "turned into fat," but it's the total number of calories you're consuming rather than the sugar in those calorie-dense foods that may contribute to new stores of fat.

◀ 14 ▶

YOUR LOW-GI FOOD FINDER

A high GI value is 70 or more.
An intermediate GI value is 56 to 69 inclusive.
A low GI value is 55 or less.

	GI VALUE				
	11–20	21–30	31–40	41–50	51–55
	11–20				
Peanut Butter	14				
Peanuts	14				
Soybeans	14				
Yogurt	14				
Fructose	19				
Maple Syrup	19				
Rice Bran	19				

	GI VALUE			
11–20	21–30	31–40	41–50	51–55

	21–30			
Cashews	22			
Cherries	22			
Choice DM Beverage, Mead Johnson	23			
Kidney Beans	23			
Barley	25			
Grapefruit	25			
Lentils	26			
Apples, Dried	29			
Prunes, Dried	29			
Black Beans	30			
Hearty Oatmeal Cookies	30			

	31–40			
Apricots, Dried		31		
Butter Beans		31		
Chocolate, Milk, Sugar-Free, FIFTY50		31		
Soy Milk		31		
Lima Beans		32		
Milk, Skim		32		
Spaghetti, Whole Wheat		32		
Split Peas, Dried		32		
M&M's Peanut		33		
Nutella		33		
Milk, Low-fat Chocolate		34		
Hearty Chocolate Meal Replacement Drink		35		
Ice Cream, Low-fat		37		
Yam		37		
All-Bran		38		

	11–20	21–30	31–40	41–50	51–55
Cannellini Beans			38		
Navy Beans			38		
Pastina			38		
Peaches, Canned			38		
Pears			38		
Rice, Converted			38		
Tomato Juice			38		
Tomato Soup			38		
Mung Beans			39		
Plums			39		
Ravioli			39		
Apple Juice			40		
Apples			40		
Fettuccine, Egg			40		
Strawberries			40		

	41–50
Bread, Pumpernickel	41
Crème-Filled Wafers, Vanilla	41
Black-eyed Peas	42
Chickpeas	42
Peaches	42
Spaghetti, Durum Wheat	42
Chocolate, Milk	43
Custard	43
Pudding	43
Lentil Soup	44
Capellini	45
Pinto Beans	45
Corn	46

		GI VALUE		
11–20	21–30	31–40	41–50	51–55

	41–50
Grapes	46
Lactose	46
Sponge Cake	46
All-Bran Bran Buds	47
Macaroni	47
Baked Beans	48
Bulgur	48
Grapefruit Juice	48
Orange Marmalade	48
Oranges	48
Peas, Green	48
Sweet Potato	48
Pears, Canned	49
Muesli	49
Oat Bran Breakfast Cereal	50
Rice, Brown	50
Tortellini, Cheese, Frozen	50

	51–55
All Bran with Extra Fiber	51
Bread, 100% Whole Grain	51
Mangoes	51
Oatmeal, Old-Fashioned	51
Strawberry Jam	51
Kidney Beans, Canned	52
Linguine, Thick	52
Spaghetti with Meat Sauce	52
Sushi	52
Bread, Sourdough Rye	53
Bread, Stone-ground 100% Whole-Wheat	53
Kiwi, Fresh	53

		GI VALUE		
11–20	21–30	31–40	41–50	51–55

	11–20	21–30	31–40	41–50	51–55
Bread, Sourdough Wheat					54
Buckwheat					54
Oatmeal Cookies					54
Pound Cake					54
Rice, Long Grain and Wild					54
Fruit Cocktail					55
Honey					55
Oat Bran, Raw					55
Semolina					55
Social Tea Biscuits					55

15

THE LOW-GI CHECKLIST

GOING GROCERY SHOPPING? Bring this list with you. It will help you choose low-GI foods quickly and easily.

BREADS

100% stoneground whole-wheat
100% stoneground whole-wheat pita
100% Whole-Grain, Natural Ovens
chapati (Baisen)
Happiness Raisin Pecan, Natural Ovens
Hearty 7 Grain, Healthy Choice
Hunger Filler, Natural Ovens
Multi-Grain Stay Trim, Natural Ovens
Natural Wheat, Natural Ovens
Nutty Natural, Natural Ovens
pumpernickel, whole-grain
rye

sourdough
sourdough rye
spelt, multigrain

BREAKFAST CEREALS

All-Bran, Kellogg's
apple and cinnamon hot cereal, ConAgra
Bran Buds with Psyllium, Kellogg's
Bran Buds, Kellogg's
Multi-Bran Chex, Kellogg's
Complete Bran flakes, Kellogg's
Just Right, Kellogg's
muesli, natural
muesli, toasted
oat bran
oat bran, raw
Raisin Bran, Kellogg's
rice bran
rolled or old-fashioned oats

COOKIES AND CAKES

Biscuits, Social Tea
bread, banana
cake, chocolate, with chocolate frosting
cake, pound
cake, sponge
cake, vanilla
cookies, Arrowroot
cookies, Hearty Oatmeal, FIFTY50

cookies, oatmeal
cookies, oatmeal, sugar free, FIFTY50
cookies, shortbread
muffin, apple cinnamon, from mix*
wafers, vanilla, cremefilled, FIFTY50

DAIRY PRODUCTS AND ALTERNATIVES

custard, homemade
ice cream, regular
milk, low-fat, chocolate, with aspartame
milk, low-fat, chocolate, with sugar
milk, skim
milk, whole
mousse, butterscotch, low-fat, Nestlé
mousse, chocolate, low-fat, Nestlé
mousse, French vanilla, low-fat, Nestlé
mousse, hazelnut, low-fat, Nestlé
mousse, mango, low-fat, Nestlé
mousse, mixed berry, low-fat, Nestlé
mousse, strawberry, low-fat, Nestlé
pudding, instant, chocolate, made with milk
pudding, instant, vanilla, made with milk
soy milk, reduced-fat
soy milk, whole
yogurt, low-fat, fruit, with aspartame
yogurt, low-fat, fruit, with sugar
yogurt, nonfat, French vanilla, with sugar
yogurt, nonfat, strawberry, with sugar

*Foods containing fat in excess of American Heart Association guidelines. Use these only once in a while and in small amounts.

FRUIT AND FRUIT PRODUCTS

apple, fresh
apricot, fresh
banana, fresh
cantaloupe, fresh
cherries, fresh
grapefruit, fresh
grapes, fresh
kiwi, fresh
mango, fresh
orange, fresh
papaya, fresh
peach, canned in natural juice
peach, fresh
pear, canned in pear juice
pear, fresh
plum, fresh
prunes, pitted
strawberries, fresh
strawberry jam

GRAINS

barley, cracked
barley, pearled
buckwheat
buckwheat groats
bulgur
rice, basmati
rice, brown
rice, Uncle Ben's Cajun Style
rice, Uncle Ben's Long Grain and Wild

rice, Uncle Ben's Converted, Original
rolled oats

JUICES

apple, with sugar or artificial sweetener
carrot, fresh
grapefruit, unsweetened
pineapple, unsweetened
tomato, canned, no added sugar

LEGUMES

beans, baked, canned
beans, butter, dried and cooked
beans, kidney, canned
beans, lima, baby, frozen
beans, mung, cooked
beans, navy, dried and cooked
beans, pinto, cooked
beans, soy, canned
chickpeas/garbanzo beans, canned
lentils, green, dried and cooked
lentils, red, dried and cooked
peas, black-eyed
peas, split, yellow, cooked

Note: Canned legumes have higher GI values than the boiled varieties because the temperatures and pressures used in the canning
process increase the digestibility of the starch. But canned
legumes are still an excellent low-fat, high-fiber, nutrient-rich low-
GI choice!

NOODLES AND PASTA

capellini
fettuccine, egg
gluten-free noodles, cornstarch
instant noodles
linguine, thick, fresh, durum wheat, white, fresh
linguine, thin, fresh, durum wheat
macaroni, plain, cooked
mung bean, Lungkow beanthread
ravioli
rice, fresh, cooked
spaghetti, cooked 22 minutes
spaghetti, cooked 5 minutes
spaghetti, protein enriched, cooked 7 minutes
spaghetti, whole wheat
spirali, cooked, durum wheat
star pastina, cooked 5 minutes
tortellini
vermicelli

SNACK FOODS

apple cinnamon snack bar, ConAgra
cashews
chocolate bar, milk, Cadbury's
chocolate bar, milk, Dove, Mars
chocolate bar, milk, Nestlé
chocolate bar, white, Milky Bar
corn chips, plain, salted, Doritos
M&M's, peanut
nougat

Nutella chocolate hazelnut spread
Peanut Butter & Chocolate Chip snack bar
peanuts
pecans
potato chips, plain, salted
Twix Cookie Bar, caramel

SOUPS

lentil, canned
minestrone, canned, ready-to-serve
tomato, canned

STARCHY VEGETABLES

corn, canned, no salt added
corn, fresh
peas
potato, new, canned
potato, sweet
yam

VEGETABLES

artichokes
avocado
bok choy
broccoli
cabbage
carrots, peeled, cooked

cassava (yucca), cooked with salt
cauliflower
celery
cucumber
French beans (runner beans)
leafy greens
lettuce
pepper
squash

Low GI Substitutes

High-GI Food	Low-GI Alternative
Bread, whole wheat or white	Bread containing a lot of whole grains such as pumpernickel or 100% stoneground whole wheat
Processed breakfast cereal	Unrefined cereal such as old-fashioned oats. Check pages 103–118 for an A-to-Z list of more than 300 other foods, and for processed cereals with low GI values (such as Kellogg's Bran Buds with Psyllium)
Cookies and crackers	Cookies made with dried fruit and whole grains such as oats
Cakes and muffins	Those made with fruit, oats, whole grains
Tropical fruits	Temperate climate fruits such as berries, apples, peaches, pears, and nectarines
Potato	New potatoes, sweet potato, yam, or substitute with corn, peas, pasta, rice, or legumes
Rice	Basmati, Uncle Ben's Original Converted, brown, or long grain rice, or substitute with barley, noodles, or pasta

Making the Change

SOME PEOPLE CHANGE their diet easily, but for the majority of us, change of any kind is difficult. Changing our diet is seldom just a matter of giving up certain foods. A healthy diet contains a wide variety of foods but we need to eat them in appropriate proportions. If you are considering changes to your diet, keep these four guidelines in mind:

1. Aim to make changes gradually.
2. Attempt the easiest changes first.
3. Break big goals into a number of smaller, more achievable goals.
4. Accept lapses in your habits.
5. If you feel like you need some extra help, seek out some professional assistance from a dietitian.

16

LET'S TALK GLYCEMIC LOAD

*I*N ADDITION TO the GI values we provide in this book, our tables also include the glycemic load (GL) value for average-sized food portions. Taken together, the glycemic index and glycemic load provide you with all the information you need to choose a diet brimming with health-boosting foods.

GLYCEMIC LOAD 101

A food's glycemic load results from the GI value and carbohydrate per serving of food. When we eat a carbohydrate-containing meal, our blood glucose first rises, then falls. The extent to which it rises and remains high is critically important to our health and depends on two things: the *amount* of a carbohydrate in the meal and the *nature* (GI value) of that carbohydrate. Both factors equally determine blood-glucose changes.

Researchers at Harvard University came up with a way of combining and describing these two factors with the term "glycemic load," which not only provides a measure of the level of glucose in the blood, but also the insulin demand produced by a normal serving of the food. Researchers measure GI values for fixed portions of foods containing a certain amount of carbohydrate (usually 50). Then, as people eat different-sized portions of the same foods, we can work out the extent to which a certain portion of food will raise the blood-glucose level by calculating a glycemic load value for that amount of food.

To calculate glycemic load, multiply a food's GI value by the amount of carbohydrate in a particular serving size, then divide by 100.

■

**Glycemic load =
(GI x carbohydrate per serving) ÷ 100**

■

For example, a small apple has a GI value of 40 and contains 15 grams of carbohydrate. Its glycemic load is (40 × 15) ÷ 100 = 6. A small 5-ounce potato has a GI value of 90 and 15 grams of carbohydrate. It has a glycemic load of (90 × 15) ÷ 100 = 14. This means one small potato will raise your blood-glucose level higher than one apple.

■

**Low GL = 10 or less
Intermediate GL = 11–19
High GL = 20 or more**

■

How GI Values Affect Glycemic Load

THE GLYCEMIC LOAD is greatest for those foods that provide the highest-GI carbohydrate, particularly those we tend to eat in large quantities. Compare the glycemic load of the following foods to see how the serving size, as well as the GI value, help to determine the glycemic response:

Rice, 1 cup	**Spaghetti, 1 cup**
Carbohydrates: 43	Carbohydrates: 40
GI: 83	GI: 44
GL: 36	GL: 18
$(83 \times 43) \div 100 = 36$	$(44 \times 40) \div 100 = 18$

Some nutritionists argue that the glycemic load is an improvement on the glycemic index because it provides an estimate of both quantity *and* quality of carbohydrate (the GI value gives us just quality) in a diet. In large Harvard studies, however, researchers were able to predict disease risk from people's overall diet, as well as its glycemic load. Using the glycemic load strengthened the relationship, suggesting that the more frequently we consume high-carbohydrate, high-GI foods, the worse it is for our health. Carbohydrate by itself has no effect—in other words, there was no benefit of low carbohydrate intake over high carbohydrate intake, or vice versa.

If you make the mistake of using GL alone, you might find yourself eating a diet with very little carbohydrate but a lot of fat and excessive amounts of protein. That's why you need to use the glycemic index to compare foods of similar nature (such as bread with bread) and use the glycemic load when you're deciding on the portion size of the carbohydrates you want to eat. If you use the technique correctly, GL values will guide you to eat smaller portions of high-GI foods.

Remember that the GL values we provide are for the standardized (nominal) portion sizes listed. If you eat a different portion size, then you'll need to calculate another GI value. Here's how: First, determine the size of your portion, then work out the available carbohydrate content of this weight (this value is listed next to the GL in our tables), then multiply by the food's GI value. For example, the nominal serving size listed for bran flakes is ½ cup, the available carbohydrate is 18 grams, and the GI value is 74. So the GL for a ½-cup serving of bran flakes is (74 × 18) ÷ 100 = 13. If, however, you normally eat 1 cup of bran flakes, you'd need to double the available carbohydrate (18 × 2 = 36) and the GL for your larger cereal portion would be (74 × 36) ÷ 100 = 27. These numbers show that the larger portion of cereal releases a larger quantity of glucose into the bloodstream.

THE TABLES

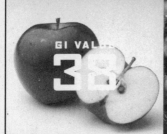

GI VALUE
38

GI VALUE
53

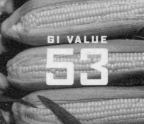

GI VALUE
29

GI VALUE
38

GI VALUE
59

GI VALUE
42

GI VALUE
46

GI VALUE
44

17
A TO Z VALUES

*T*HE TABLE IN this section will help you find a food's glycemic index value quickly and easily, because we've listed the foods alphabetically.

The list provides not only the food's GI value but also its glycemic load (see Chapter 16). We calculate the glycemic load using a nominal, or standardized, serving size as well as the carbohydrate content of that serving—both of which we've also listed. That way, you can choose foods with either a low GI value or a low glycemic load. If your favorite food is both high-GI and high-GL, you can either cut down the serving size or dilute the GL by combining it with very low-GI foods, such as rice and lentils.

For the first time, we've also included foods that have very little carbohydrate; their GI value is zero, indicated by [0]. Many vegetables, such as avocados and broccoli, and protein foods such as chicken, cheese, and tuna, fall into the low- or no-carbohydrate category. Most alcoholic beverages are also low in carbohydrate.

Key to the Table

GI: The glycemic index value for the food, where glucose equals 100

Nominal Serving Size: The portion of food tested

Net Carb per Serving: The total grams of carbohydrates available to the body for digestion from the particular food in the specific serving size (total grams of carbs minus grams of fiber)

GL per Serving: Glycemic load of the food; this relates to the quantity of carbohydrates that will enter the bloodstream for the particular food in the specific serving size

FOOD	GI Value	Nominal Serving Size	Net Carb per Serving	GL per Serving
A				
All-Bran, breakfast cereal	30	½ cup	15	4
Almonds	[0]	1.75 oz	0	0
Angel food cake, 1 slice	67	¹⁄₁₂ cake	29	19
Apple, dried	29	9 rings	34	10
Apple, fresh, medium	38	4 oz	15	6
Apple juice, pure, unsweetened, reconstituted	40	8 oz	29	12
Apple muffin, small	44	3.5 oz	41	18
Apricots, canned in light syrup	64	4 halves	19	12
Apricots, dried	30	17 halves	27	8
Apricots, fresh, 3 medium	57	4 oz	9	5
Arborio, risotto rice, cooked	69	¾ cup	53	36
Artichokes (Jerusalem)	[0]	½ cup	0	0
Avocado	[0]	¼	0	0
B				
Bagel, white	72	½	35	25
Baked beans	38	⅔ cup	31	12
Baked beans, canned in tomato sauce	48	⅔ cup	15	7
Banana cake, 1 slice	47	⅛ cake	38	18
Banana, fresh, medium	52	4 oz	24	12
Barley, pearled, cooked	25	1 cup	42	11
Basmati rice, white, cooked	58	1 cup	38	22
Beef	[0]	4 oz	0	0
Beer	[0]	8 oz	10	0
Beets, canned	64	½ cup	7	5
Bengal gram dahl, chickpea	11	5 oz	36	4
Black bean soup	64	1 cup	27	17
Black beans, cooked	30	⅘ cup	23	7
Black-eyed peas, canned	42	⅔ cup	17	7

[0] indicates that the food has so little carbohydrate that the GI value cannot be tested. The GL, therefore, is 0.

FOOD	GI Value	Nominal Serving Size	Net Carb per Serving	GL per Serving
Blueberry muffin, small	59	3.5 oz	47	28
Bok choy, raw	[0]	1 cup	0	0
Bran Flakes, breakfast cereal	74	½ cup	18	13
Bran muffin, small	60	3.5 oz	41	25
Brandy	[0]	1 oz	0	0
Brazil nuts	[0]	1.75 oz	0	0
Breton wheat crackers	67	6	14	10
Broad beans	79	½ cup	11	9
Broccoli, raw	[0]	1 cup	0	0
Broken rice, white, cooked	86	1 cup	43	37
Brown rice, cooked	50	1 cup	33	16
Buckwheat	54	¾ cup	30	16
Bulgur, cooked 20 min	48	¾ cup	26	12
Bun, hamburger	61	1.5 oz	22	13
Butter beans, canned	31	⅔ cup	20	6

C

FOOD	GI Value	Nominal Serving Size	Net Carb per Serving	GL per Serving
Cabbage, raw	[0]	1 cup	0	0
Cactus Nectar, Organic Agave, light, 90% fructose (Western Commerce)	11	1 Tbsp	8	1
Cactus Nectar, Organic Agave, light, 97% fructose (Western Commerce)	10	1 Tbsp	8	1
Cantaloupe, fresh	65	4 oz	6	4
Cappellini pasta, cooked	45	1½ cups	45	20
Carrot juice, fresh	43	8 oz	23	10
Carrots, peeled, cooked	49	½ cup	5	2
Carrots, raw	47	1 medium	6	3
Cashew nuts, salted	22	1.75 oz	13	3
Cauliflower, raw	[0]	¾ cup	0	0
Celery, raw	[0]	2 stalks	0	0
Cheese	[0]	4 oz	0	0

[0] indicates that the food has so little carbohydrate that the GI value cannot be tested. The GL, therefore, is 0.

FOOD	GI Value	Nominal Serving Size	Net Carb per Serving	GL per Serving
Cherries, fresh	22	18	12	3
Chicken nuggets, frozen	46	4 oz	16	7
Chickpeas, canned	42	⅔ cup	22	9
Chickpeas, dried, cooked	28	⅔ cup	30	8
Chocolate cake made from mix with chocolate frosting	38	4 oz	52	20
Chocolate milk, low-fat	34	8 oz	26	9
Chocolate mousse, 2% fat	31	½ cup	22	7
Chocolate powder, dissolved in water	55	8 oz	16	9
Chocolate pudding, made from powder and whole milk	47	½ cup	24	11
Choice DM, nutritional support product, vanilla (Mead Johnson)	23	8 oz	24	6
Clif bar (cookies & cream)	101	2.4 oz	34	34
Coca Cola, soft drink	53	8 oz	26	14
Cocoa Puffs, breakfast cereal	77	1 cup	26	20
Complete, breakfast cereal	48	1 cup	21	10
Condensed milk, sweetened	61	2½ Tbsps	27	17
Converted rice, long-grain, cooked 20–30 min, Uncle Ben's	50	1 cup	36	18
Converted rice, white, cooked 20–30 min, Uncle Ben's	38	1 cup	36	14
Corn Flakes, breakfast cereal	92	1 cup	26	24
Corn Flakes, Honey Crunch, breakfast cereal	72	¾ cup	25	18
Corn pasta, gluten-free	78	1¼ cups	42	32
Corn Pops, breakfast cereal	80	1 cup	26	21
Corn Thins, puffed corn cakes, gluten-free	87	1 oz	20	18
Corn, sweet, cooked	60	½ cup	18	11
Cornmeal, cooked 2 min	68	1 cup	13	9
Couscous, cooked 5 min	65	¾ cup	35	23

[0] indicates that the food has so little carbohydrate that the GI value cannot be tested. The GL, therefore, is 0.

FOOD	GI Value	Nominal Serving Size	Net Carb per Serving	GL per Serving
Cranberry juice cocktail	52	8 oz	31	16
Crispix, breakfast cereal	87	1 cup	25	22
Croissant, medium	67	2 oz	26	17
Cucumber, raw	[0]	¾ cup	0	0
Cupcake, strawberry-iced, small	73	1.5 oz	26	19
Custard apple, raw, flesh only	54	4 oz	19	10
Custard, homemade	43	½ cup	26	11
Custard, prepared from powder with whole milk, instant	35	½ cup	26	9

D

FOOD	GI Value	Nominal Serving Size	Net Carb per Serving	GL per Serving
Dates, dried	50	7	40	20
Desiree potato, peeled, cooked	101	5 oz	17	17
Doughnut, cake type	76	1.75 oz	23	17

E

FOOD	GI Value	Nominal Serving Size	Net Carb per Serving	GL per Serving
Eggs, large	[0]	2	0	0
Enercal Plus (Wyeth-Ayerst)	61	8 oz	40	24
English Muffin bread (Natural Ovens)	77	1 oz	14	11
Ensure, vanilla drink	48	8 oz	34	16
Ensure bar, chocolate fudge brownie	43	1.4 oz	20	8
Ensure Plus, vanilla drink	40	8 oz	47	19
Ensure Pudding, old-fashioned vanilla	36	4 oz	26	9

F

FOOD	GI Value	Nominal Serving Size	Net Carb per Serving	GL per Serving
Fanta, orange soft drink	68	8 oz	34	23
Fettuccine, egg, cooked	32	1½ cups	46	15
Figs, dried	61	3	26	16
Fish	[0]	4 oz	0	0
Fish sticks	38	3.5 oz	19	7
Flan/crème caramel	65	½ cup	73	47
French baguette, white, plain	95	1 oz	15	15

[0] indicates that the food has so little carbohydrate that the GI value cannot be tested. The GL, therefore, is 0.

FOOD	GI Value	Nominal Serving Size	Net Carb per Serving	GL per Serving
French fries, frozen, reheated in microwave	75	30 pcs	29	22
French green beans, cooked	[0]	½ cup	0	0
French vanilla cake made from mix, with vanilla frosting	42	4 oz	58	24
French vanilla ice cream, premium, 16% fat	38	½ cup	14	5
Froot Loops, breakfast cereal	69	1 cup	26	18
Frosted Flakes, breakfast cereal	55	1 cup	26	15
Fructose, pure	19	1 Tbsp	10	2
Fruit cocktail, canned, light syrup	55	½ cup	16	9
Fruit leather	61	2 pcs	24	15
G				
Gatorade (orange) sports drink	89	8 oz	15	13
Gin	[0]	1 oz	0	0
Glucerna, vanilla (Abbott)	31	8 oz	23	7
Glucose (dextrose)	99	1 Tbsp	10	10
Glucose tablets	102	3 pcs	15	15
Gluten-free corn pasta	78	1½ cups	42	32
Gluten-free multigrain bread	79	1 oz	13	10
Gluten-free rice and corn pasta	76	1½ cups	49	37
Gluten-free spaghetti, rice and split pea, canned in tomato sauce	68	8 oz	27	19
Gluten-free split pea and soy pasta shells	29	1½ cups	31	9
Gluten-free white bread, sliced	80	1 oz	15	12
Glutinous (sticky) rice, white, cooked	92	⅔ cup	48	44
Gnocchi	68	6 oz	48	33
Grapefruit, fresh, medium	25	1 half	11	3
Grapefruit juice, unsweetened	48	8 oz	20	9
Grape-Nuts, breakfast cereal (Post)	75	¼ cup	21	16

[0] indicates that the food has so little carbohydrate that the GI value cannot be tested. The GL, therefore, is 0.

FOOD	GI Value	Nominal Serving Size	Net Carb per Serving	GL per Serving
Grapes, black, fresh	59	¾ cup	18	11
Grapes, green, fresh	46	¾ cup	18	8
Green peas	48	⅓ cup	7	3
Green pea soup, canned	66	8 oz	41	27
H				
Hamburger bun	61	1.5 oz	22	13
Happiness (cinnamon, raisin, pecan bread) (Natural Ovens)	63	1 oz	14	9
Hazelnuts	[0]	1.75 oz	0	0
Healthy Choice Hearty 100% Whole Grain	62	1 oz	14	9
Healthy Choice Hearty 7 Grain	55	1 oz	14	8
Hearty Oatmeal cookies	30	4	20	6
Honey	55	1 Tbsp	18	10
Hot cereal, apple & cinnamon, dry (ConAgra)	37	1.2 oz	22	8
Hot cereal, unflavored, dry (ConAgra)	25	1.2 oz	19	5
Hunger Filler, whole-grain bread (Natural Ovens)	59	1 oz	13	7
I				
Ice cream, low-fat, vanilla, "light"	50	½ cup	9	5
Ice cream, premium, French vanilla, 16% fat	38	½ cup	14	5
Ice cream, premium, "ultra chocolate," 15% fat	37	½ cup	14	5
Ice cream, regular fat	61	½ cup	20	12
Instant potato, mashed	97	¾ cup	20	17
Instant rice, white, cooked 6 min	87	¾ cup	42	36
Ironman PR bar, chocolate	39	2.3 oz	26	10

[0] indicates that the food has so little carbohydrate that the GI value cannot be tested. The GL, therefore, is 0.

FOOD	GI Value	Nominal Serving Size	Net Carb per Serving	GL per Serving
J				
Jam, apricot fruit spread, reduced sugar	55	1½ Tbsps	13	7
Jam, strawberry	51	1½ Tbsps	20	10
Jasmine rice, white, cooked	109	1 cup	42	46
Jelly beans	78	10 large	28	22
K				
Kaiser roll	73	1 half	16	12
Kavli™ Norwegian crispbread	71	5 pcs	16	12
Kidney beans, canned	52	⅔ cup	17	9
Kidney beans, dried, cooked	23	⅔ cup	25	6
Kiwi fruit	53	4 oz	12	7
Kudos Whole Grain Bars, chocolate chip	62	1.8 oz	32	20
L				
Lactose, pure	46	1 Tbsp	10	5
Lamb	[0]	4 oz	0	0
Leafy vegetables (spinach, arugula, etc.), raw	[0]	1½ cups	0	0
L.E.A.N Fibergy bar, Harvest Oat	45	1.75 oz	29	13
L.E.A.N Life long Nutribar, Chocolate Crunch	32	1.5 oz	19	6
L.E.A.N Life long Nutribar, Peanut Crunch	30	1.5 oz	19	6
L.E.A.N Nutrimeal, drink powder, Dutch Chocolate	26	8 oz	13	3
Lemonade, reconstituted	66	8 oz	20	13
Lentil soup, canned	44	9 oz	21	9
Lentils, brown, cooked	29	¾ cup	18	5
Lentils, green, cooked	30	¾ cup	17	5
Lentils, red, cooked	26	¾ cup	18	5

[0] indicates that the food has so little carbohydrate that the GI value cannot be tested. The GL, therefore, is 0.

FOOD	GI Value	Nominal Serving Size	Net Carb per Serving	GL per Serving
Lettuce	[0]	4 leaves	0	0
Life Savers, peppermint candy	70	18 pcs	30	21
Light rye bread	68	1 oz	14	10
Lima beans, baby, frozen	32	¾ cup	30	10
Linguine pasta, thick, cooked	46	1½ cups	48	22
Linguine pasta, thin, cooked	52	1½ cups	45	23
Long-grain rice, cooked 10 min	61	1 cup	36	22
Lychees, canned in syrup, drained	79	4 oz	20	16
M				
M & M's, peanut	33	15 pcs	17	6
Macadamia nuts	[0]	1.75 oz	0	0
Macaroni and cheese, made from mix	64	1 cup	51	32
Macaroni, cooked	47	1¼ cups	48	23
Maltose	105	1 Tbsp	10	11
Mango	51	4 oz	15	8
Maple syrup, pure Canadian	54	1 Tbsp	18	10
Marmalade, orange	48	1½ Tbsps	20	9
Mars Bar	68	2 oz	40	27
Melba toast, Old London	70	6 pcs	23	16
METRx bar (vanilla)	74	3.6 oz	50	37
Milk Arrowroot cookies	69	5	18	12
Millet, cooked	71	⅔ cup	36	25
Mini Wheats, whole-wheat breakfast cereal	58	12 pcs	21	12
Mousse, butterscotch, 1.9% fat	36	1.75 oz	10	4
Mousse, chocolate, 2% fat	31	1.75 oz	11	3
Mousse, hazelnut, 2.4% fat	36	1.75 oz	10	4
Mousse, mango, 1.8% fat	33	1.75 oz	11	4
Mousse, mixed berry, 2.2% fat	36	1.75 oz	10	4
Mousse, strawberry, 2.3% fat	32	1.75 oz	10	3

[0] indicates that the food has so little carbohydrate that the GI value cannot be tested. The GL, therefore, is 0.

FOOD	GI Value	Nominal Serving Size	Net Carb per Serving	GL per Serving
Muesli bar containing dried fruit	61	1 oz	21	13
Muesli bread, made from mix in bread oven (ConAgra)	54	1 oz	12	7
Muesli, gluten-free, with low-fat milk	39	1 oz	19	7
Muesli, Swiss Formula	56	1 oz	16	9
Muesli, toasted	43	1 oz	17	7
Multi-Grain 9-Grain bread	43	1 oz	14	6
N				
Navy beans, canned	38	5 oz	31	12
Nesquik, chocolate dissolved in low-fat milk, no-sugar-added	41	8 oz	11	5
Nesquik, strawberry dissolved in low-fat milk, no-sugar-added	35	8 oz	12	4
New creamer potato, canned	65	5 oz	18	12
New creamer potato, unpeeled and cooked 20 min	78	5 oz	21	16
Noodles, instant "two-minute" (Maggi)	46	1½ cups	40	19
Noodles, mung bean (Lungkow beanthread), dried, cooked	39	1½ cups	45	18
Noodles, rice, fresh, cooked	40	1½ cups	39	15
Nutella, chocolate hazelnut spread	33	1 Tbsp	12	4
Nutrigrain, breakfast cereal	66	1 cup	15	10
Nutty Natural, whole-grain bread (Natural Ovens)	59	1 oz	12	7
O				
Oat bran, raw	55	2 Tbsp	5	3
Oatmeal, cooked 1 min	66	1 cup	26	17
Oatmeal cookies	55	4 small	21	12
Oatmeal cookies, Sugar-Free (FIFTY50)	47	4	28	10

[0] indicates that the food has so little carbohydrate that the GI value cannot be tested. The GL, therefore, is 0.

FOOD	GI Value	Nominal Serving Size	Net Carb per Serving	GL per Serving
Orange juice, unsweetened, reconstituted	53	8 oz	18	9
Orange, fresh, medium	42	4 oz	11	5
P				
Pancakes, buckwheat, gluten-free, made from mix	102	2 4"-round	22	22
Pancakes, made from mix	67	2 4"-round	58	39
Papaya, fresh	59	4 oz	8	5
Parsnips	97	½ cup	12	12
Pastry	59	2 oz	26	15
Pea soup, canned	66	8 oz	41	27
Peach, canned in heavy syrup	58	½ cup	26	15
Peach, canned in light syrup	52	½ cup	18	9
Peach, fresh, large	42	4 oz	11	5
Peanuts	14	1.75 oz	6	1
Pear halves, canned in natural juice	43	½ cup	13	5
Pear, fresh	38	4 oz	11	4
Peas, green, frozen, cooked	48	½ cup	7	3
Pecans	[0]	1.75 oz	0	0
Pepper, fresh, green or red	[0]	3 oz	0	0
Pineapple, fresh	66	4 oz	10	6
Pineapple juice, unsweetened	46	8 oz	34	15
Pinto beans, canned	45	⅔ cup	22	10
Pinto beans, dried, cooked	39	¾ cup	26	10
Pita bread, white	57	1 oz	17	10
Pizza, cheese	60	1 slice	27	16
Pizza, Super Supreme, pan, 11.4% fat	36	1 slice	24	9
Pizza, Super Supreme, thin and crispy, 13.2% fat	30	1 slice	22	7
Plums, fresh	39	2 medium	12	5
Pop Tarts, double chocolate	70	1.8 oz	36	25

[0] indicates that the food has so little carbohydrate that the GI value cannot be tested. The GL, therefore, is 0.

FOOD	GI Value	Nominal Serving Size	Net Carb per Serving	GL per Serving
Popcorn, plain, cooked in microwave oven	72	1½ cups	11	8
Pork	[0]	4 oz	0	0
Potato chips, plain, salted	54	2 oz	21	11
Potato, baked	85	5 oz	30	26
Potato, microwaved	82	5 oz	33	27
Pound cake (Sara Lee)	54	2 oz	28	15
PowerBar, chocolate	57	2.3 oz	42	24
Premium soda crackers	74	5	17	12
Pretzels	83	1 oz	20	16
Prunes, pitted	29	6	33	10
Pudding, instant, chocolate, made with whole milk	47	½ cup	24	11
Pudding, instant, vanilla, made with whole milk	40	½ cup	24	10
Puffed crispbread	81	1 oz	19	15
Puffed rice cakes, white	82	3	21	17
Puffed Wheat, breakfast cereal	80	2 cups	21	17
Pumpernickel rye kernel bread	41	1 oz	12	5
Pumpkin	75	3 oz	4	3

R

FOOD	GI Value	Nominal Serving Size	Net Carb per Serving	GL per Serving
Raisin Bran, breakfast cereal	61	½ cup	19	12
Raisins	64	½ cup	44	28
Ravioli, meat-filled, cooked	39	6.5 oz	38	15
Red wine	[0]	3.5 oz	0	0
Red-skinned potato, peeled and microwaved on high for 6–7.5 min	79	5 oz	18	14
Red-skinned potato, peeled, boiled 35 min	88	5 oz	18	16
Red-skinned potato, peeled, mashed	91	5 oz	20	18

[0] indicates that the food has so little carbohydrate that the GI value cannot be tested. The GL, therefore, is 0.

FOOD	GI Value	Nominal Serving Size	Net Carb per Serving	GL per Serving
Resource Diabetic, nutritional support product, vanilla (Novartis)	34	8 oz	23	8
Rice and corn pasta, gluten-free	76	1½ cups	49	37
Rice bran, extruded	19	1 oz	14	3
Rice cakes, white	82	3	21	17
Rice Krispies, breakfast cereal	82	1¼ cups	26	22
Rice Krispies Treat bar	63	1 oz	24	15
Rice noodles, fresh, cooked	40	1½ cups	39	15
Rice, parboiled	72	1 cup	36	26
Rice pasta, brown, cooked 16 min	92	1½ cups	38	35
Rice vermicelli	58	1½ cups	39	22
Rolled oats	42	1 cup	21	9
Roll-Ups, processed fruit snack	99	1 oz	25	24
Roman (cranberry) beans, fresh, cooked	46	¾ cup	18	8
Russet, baked potato	85	5 oz	30	26
Rutabaga, fresh, cooked	72	5 oz	10	7
Rye bread	58	1 oz	14	8
Ryvita crackers	69	3	16	11
S				
Salami	[0]	4 oz	0	0
Salmon	[0]	4 oz	0	0
Sausages, fried	28	3.5 oz	3	1
Scones, plain	92	1 oz	9	8
Sebago potato, peeled, cooked	87	5 oz	17	14
Seeded rye bread	55	1 oz	13	7
Semolina, cooked (dry)	55	⅓ cup	50	28
Shellfish (shrimp, crab, lobster, etc.)	[0]	4 oz	0	0
Sherry	[0]	2 oz	0	0
Shortbread cookies	64	1 oz	16	10

[0] indicates that the food has so little carbohydrate that the GI value cannot be tested. The GL, therefore, is 0.

FOOD	GI Value	Nominal Serving Size	Net Carb per Serving	GL per Serving
Shredded Wheat, breakfast cereal	75	⅔ cup	20	15
Shredded Wheat biscuits	62	1 oz	18	11
Skim milk	32	8 oz	13	4
Skittles	70	45 pcs	45	32
Smacks, breakfast cereal	71	¾ cup	23	11
Smoothie, raspberry (ConAgra)	33	8 oz	41	14
Snack bar, Apple Cinnamon (ConAgra)	40	1.75 oz	29	12
Snack bar, Peanut Butter & Choc-Chip (ConAgra)	37	1.75 oz	27	10
Snickers bar	68	2.2 oz	35	23
Soda crackers, Premium	74	5	17	12
Soft drink, Coca Cola	53	8 oz	26	14
Soft drink, Fanta, orange	68	8 oz	34	23
Sourdough rye	48	1 oz	12	6
Sourdough wheat	54	1 oz	14	8
Soy & Flaxseed bread (mix in bread oven) (ConAgra)	50	1 oz	10	5
Soybeans, canned	14	1 cup	6	1
Soybeans, dried, cooked	20	1 cup	6	1
Spaghetti, durum wheat, cooked 20 min	64	1½ cups	43	27
Spaghetti, gluten-free, rice and split pea, canned in tomato sauce	68	8 oz	27	19
Spaghetti, white, cooked 5 min	38	1½ cups	48	18
Spaghetti, whole wheat, cooked 5 min	32	1½ cups	44	14
Special K, breakfast cereal	69	1 cup	21	14
Spirali pasta, durum wheat, al dente	43	1½ cups	44	19
Split pea and soy pasta shells, gluten-free	29	1½ cups	31	9
Split-pea soup	60	1 cup	27	16
Split peas, yellow, cooked 20 min	32	¾ cup	19	6

[0] indicates that the food has so little carbohydrate that the GI value cannot be tested. The GL, therefore, is 0.

FOOD	GI Value	Nominal Serving Size	Net Carb per Serving	GL per Serving
Sponge cake, plain	46	2 oz	36	17
Squash, raw	[0]	⅔ cup	0	0
Star pastina, white, cooked 5 min	38	1½ cups	48	18
Stay Trim, whole-grain bread (Natural Ovens)	70	1 oz	15	10
Stoned Wheat Thins	67	14 crackers	17	12
Strawberries, fresh	40	4 oz	3	1
Strawberry jam	51	1½ Tbsps	20	10
Strawberry shortcake	42	2.2 oz	40	17
Stuffing, bread	74	1 oz	21	16
Sucrose	68	1 Tbsp	10	7
Super Supreme pizza, pan, 11.4% fat	36	1 slice	24	9
Super Supreme pizza, thin and crispy, 13.2% fat	30	1 slice	22	7
Sushi, salmon	48	3.5 oz	36	17
Sweet corn, whole kernel, canned, diet-pack, drained	46	1 cup	28	13
Sweet potato, cooked	44	5 oz	25	11

T

FOOD	GI Value	Nominal Serving Size	Net Carb per Serving	GL per Serving
Taco shells, baked	68	2	12	8
Tapioca, cooked with milk	81	¾ cup	18	14
Tofu-based frozen dessert, chocolate with high-fructose (24%) corn syrup	115	1.75 oz	9	10
Tomato juice, canned, no added sugar	38	8 oz	9	4
Tomato soup	38	1 cup	17	6
Tortellini, cheese	50	6.5 oz	21	10
Tortilla chips, plain, salted	63	1.75 oz	26	17
Total, breakfast cereal	76	¾ cup	22	17
Tuna	[0]	4 oz	0	0
Twix Cookie Bar, caramel	44	2	39	17

[0] indicates that the food has so little carbohydrate that the GI value cannot be tested. The GL, therefore, is 0.

FOOD	GI Value	Nominal Serving Size	Net Carb per Serving	GL per Serving
U				
Ultra chocolate ice cream, premium, 15% fat	37	½ cup	14	5
Ultracal with fiber (Mead Johnson)	40	8 oz	29	12
V				
Vanilla cake made from mix, with vanilla frosting	42	4 oz	58	24
Vanilla pudding, instant, made with whole milk	40	½ cup	24	10
Vanilla wafers, creme-filled (Fifty50)	41	4 cookies	20	8
Vanilla wafers	77	6 cookies	18	14
Veal	[0]	4 oz	0	0
Vermicelli, white, cooked	35	1½ cups	44	16
W				
Waffles, Aunt Jemima	76	1 4" waffle	13	10
Walnuts	[0]	1.75 oz	0	0
Water crackers	78	7	18	14
Watermelon, fresh	72	4 oz	6	4
Weet-Bix, breakfast cereal	69	2 biscuits	17	12
Wheaties, breakfast cereal	82	1 cup	21	17
Whiskey	[0]	1 oz	0	0
White bread	70	1 oz	14	10
White rice, instant, cooked 6 min	87	1 cup	42	36
White wine	[0]	3.5 oz	0	0
100% Whole Grain bread (Natural Ovens)	51	1 oz	13	7
Whole milk	31	8 oz	12	4
Whole-wheat bread	77	1 oz	12	9
Wonder white bread	80	1 oz	14	11

[0] indicates that the food has so little carbohydrate that the GI value cannot be tested. The GL, therefore, is 0.

FOOD	GI Value	Nominal Serving Size	Net Carb per Serving	GL per Serving
X				
Xylitol	8	1 Tbsp	10	1
Y				
Yam, peeled, cooked	37	5 oz	36	13
Yogurt, low-fat, wild strawberry	31	8 oz	34	11
Yogurt, low-fat, with fruit and artificial sweetener	14	8 oz	15	2
Yogurt, low-fat, with fruit and sugar	33	8 oz	35	12

[0] indicates that the food has so little carbohydrate that the GI value cannot be tested. The GL, therefore, is 0.

◀ 18 ▶

LOW TO HIGH GI VALUES

$\mathcal{F}$OR THOSE WHO wish to choose a diet with the lowest GI values possible, we've created the following listing in order of GI values (i.e., from lowest to highest value). We've also divided the list into food categories, so that when you want to find a low-GI vegetable or fruit, for example, the information is at your fingertips. The categories are:

- bakery products
- beverages
- breads
- breakfast foods
- cookies
- crackers
- dairy products and alternatives
- fruits and fruit products
- grains
- infant formulas and baby foods

- legumes
- meal-replacement products
- mixed meals and convenience foods
- noodles
- pasta
- protein foods
- snack foods and candy
- soups
- special dietary products
- sugars
- vegetables

As we discuss in *The New Glucose Revolution,* it's not necessary to eat all of your carbohydrates from low-GI sources. If half of your carbohydrate choices have low GI values, you're doing well. If you also eat a low-GI food at each meal, you'll be reducing the GI values overall.

FOOD	LOW	INTERMEDIATE	HIGH

BAKERY PRODUCTS

Cakes

Food	LOW	INTERMEDIATE	HIGH
Banana	○		
Chocolate, with chocolate frosting	○		
Pound	○		
Sponge	○		
Vanilla	○		
Angel food		◑	
Flan		◑	

Muffins

Food	LOW	INTERMEDIATE	HIGH
Apple with sugar or artificial sweeteners	○		
Apple, oat, and raisin	○		
Banana, oat, and honey		◑	
Bran		◑	
Blueberry		◑	
Carrot		◑	
Oatmeal, made from mix, Quaker Oats		◑	
Cupcake, iced			●
Scone, plain			●

Pastries

Food	LOW	INTERMEDIATE	HIGH
Croissant		◑	
Doughnut, cake-type			●

BEVERAGES

Alcoholic

Food	LOW	INTERMEDIATE	HIGH
Beer	○		
Brandy	○		

FOOD	LOW	INTERMEDIATE	HIGH
Gin	○		
Sherry	○		
Whiskey	○		
Wine, red	○		
Wine, white	○		
Juices			
Apple, with sugar or artificial sweetener	○		
Carrot, fresh	○		
Grapefruit, unsweetened	○		
Pineapple, unsweetened	○		
Tomato, canned, no added sugar	○		
Smoothies and Shakes			
Raspberry	○		
Soy	○		
Soft drinks			
Coca-Cola		◐	
Fanta		◐	
Sports drinks			
Gatorade			●

BREADS

Fruit			
Muesli, made from mix	○		
Natural Ovens Happiness, cinnamon, raisin, pecan		◐	
Gluten-free			
Fiber-enriched			●
White			●

FOOD	LOW	INTERMEDIATE	HIGH
Rye			
Pumpernickel	◯		
Sourdough	◯		
Cocktail		◑	
Light		◑	
Whole wheat		◑	
Spelt			
Multigrain	◯		
White			●
Wheat			
100% Whole Grain	◯		
Soy & Linseed bread machine mix	◯		
Flatbread, Indian		◑	
Hearty 7 Grain		◑	
Pita, plain		◑	
Bagel			●
Baguette			●
Bread stuffing			●
English Muffin			●
Flatbread, Middle Eastern			●
Italian			●
Lebanese, white			●
White, enriched			●
Whole wheat			●

FOOD	LOW	INTERMEDIATE	HIGH

BREAKFAST FOODS

Breakfast cereal bars

FOOD	LOW	INTERMEDIATE	HIGH
Rice Krispies Treat		◖	

Cooked cereals

FOOD	LOW	INTERMEDIATE	HIGH
Hot cereal, apple & cinnamon, ConAgra	○		
Old-fashioned oats	○		
Cream of Wheat, regular, Nabisco		◖	
One Minute Oats, Quaker Oats		◖	
Quick Oats, Quaker Oats		◖	
Cream of Wheat, instant, Nabisco			●
Oatmeal, instant			●

Grain products

FOOD	LOW	INTERMEDIATE	HIGH
Pancakes, prepared from mix	○		
Pancakes, buckwheat, gluten-free, made from mix			●
Waffles, Aunt Jemima			●

Ready-to-eat cereals

FOOD	LOW	INTERMEDIATE	HIGH
All-Bran, Kellogg's	○		
Complete Bran Flakes, Kellogg's	○		
Bran Buds, Kellogg's		◖	
Bran Chex, Kellogg's		◖	
Froot Loops, Kellogg's		◖	
Frosted Flakes, Kellogg's		◖	
Just Right, Kellogg's		◖	
Life, Quaker Oats		◖	
Nutrigrain, Kellogg's		◖	
Oat bran, raw, Quaker Oats		◖	
Puffed Wheat, Quaker Oats		◖	

FOOD	LOW	INTERMEDIATE	HIGH
Raisin Bran, Kellogg's		◑	
Special K, Kellogg's		◑	
Bran Flakes, Kellogg's			●
Cheerios, General Mills			●
Corn Chex, Kellogg's			●
Corn Flakes, Kellogg's			●
Corn Pops, Kellogg's			●
Grapenuts, Post			●
Rice Krispies, Kellogg's			●
Shredded Wheat, Nabisco			●
Team Flakes, Nabisco			●
Total			●
Weetabix			●

COOKIES

FOOD	LOW	INTERMEDIATE	HIGH
Hearty Oatmeal, FIFTY50	○		
Oatmeal, Sugar-Free, FIFTY50	○		
Vanilla wafers, creme filled, FIFTY50	○		
Arrowroot		◑	
Digestives		◑	
Tea biscuits		◑	
Shortbread		◑	
Vanilla wafers			●

CRACKERS

FOOD	LOW	INTERMEDIATE	HIGH
Breton wheat		◑	
Melba toast		◑	
Rye crispbread		◑	
Ryvita		◑	
Stoned Wheat Thins		◑	

FOOD	LOW	INTERMEDIATE	HIGH
Water		◐	
Kavli Norwegian Crispbread			●
Premium soda (Saltines)			●
Rice cakes, puffed			●

DAIRY PRODUCTS AND ALTERNATIVES

Custard

	LOW	INTERMEDIATE	HIGH
Homemade	○		

Ice cream

	LOW	INTERMEDIATE	HIGH
Regular	○		

Milk

	LOW	INTERMEDIATE	HIGH
Low-fat, chocolate, with aspartame	○		
Low-fat, chocolate, with sugar	○		
Skim	○		
Whole	○		
Condensed, sweetened			●

Mousse

	LOW	INTERMEDIATE	HIGH
Butterscotch, low-fat, Nestlé	○		
Chocolate, low-fat, Nestlé	○		
French vanilla, low-fat, Nestlé	○		
Hazelnut, low-fat, Nestlé	○		
Mango, low-fat, Nestlé	○		
Mixed berry, low-fat, Nestlé	○		
Strawberry, low-fat, Nestlé	○		

Pudding

	LOW	INTERMEDIATE	HIGH
Instant, chocolate, made with milk	○		
Instant, vanilla, made with milk	○		

FOOD	LOW	INTERMEDIATE	HIGH
Soy milk			
Reduced fat	○		
Whole	○		
Soy yogurt			
Tofu-based frozen dessert, chocolate			●
Yogurt			
Low-fat, fruit, with aspartame	○		
Low-fat, fruit, with sugar	○		
Nonfat, French vanilla, with sugar	○		
Nonfat, strawberry, with sugar	○		

FRUIT AND FRUIT PRODUCTS

FOOD	LOW	INTERMEDIATE	HIGH
Apple, fresh	○		
Apricot, fresh	○		
Banana, fresh	○		
Cantaloupe, fresh	○		
Cherries, fresh	○		
Grapefruit, fresh	○		
Grapes, fresh	○		
Mango, fresh	○		
Orange, fresh	○		
Peach, canned in natural juice	○		
Peach, fresh	○		
Pear, canned in pear juice	○		
Pear, fresh	○		
Plum, fresh	○		
Prunes, pitted	○		
Strawberries, fresh	○		
Strawberry jam	○		
Figs, dried		◑	
Fruit cocktail, canned		◑	

FOOD	LOW	INTERMEDIATE	HIGH
Kiwi, fresh	◑		
Papaya, fresh		◑	
Peach, canned in heavy syrup		◑	
Peach, canned in light syrup		◑	
Pineapple, fresh		◑	
Raisins/sultanas		◑	
Dates, dried			●
Lychee, canned in syrup, drained			●
Watermelon, fresh			●

GRAINS

FOOD	LOW	INTERMEDIATE	HIGH
Barley, cracked	○		
Barley, pearled	○		
Buckwheat	○		
Buckwheat groats	○		
Bulgur	○		
Corn, canned, no salt added	○		
Rice, brown	○		
Rice, Cajun Style, Uncle Ben's	○		
Rice, Long Grain and Wild, Uncle Ben's	○		
Rice, parboiled, converted, white, cooked 20–30 min, Uncle Ben's	○		
Barley, rolled		◑	
Corn, fresh		◑	
Cornmeal		◑	
Couscous		◑	
Rice, arborio (risotto)		◑	
Rice, Basmati		◑	
Rice, Garden Style, Uncle Ben's		◑	
Rice, parboiled, long grain, cooked 10 minutes		◑	
Millet			●

FOOD	LOW	INTERMEDIATE	HIGH
Rice, sticky			●
Rice, parboiled			●
Tapioca boiled with milk			●

INFANT FORMULA AND BABY FOODS

Baby foods

FOOD	LOW	INTERMEDIATE	HIGH
Apple, apricot, and banana, baby cereal		◑	
Chicken and noodles with vegetables, strained		◑	
Corn and rice, baby		◑	
Oatmeal, creamed, baby		◑	
Rice pudding, baby		◑	

Infant formula

FOOD	LOW	INTERMEDIATE	HIGH
SMA, 20 cal/fl oz, Wyeth	○		
Nursoy, soy-based, milk-free, Wyeth		◑	

LEGUMES

Beans

FOOD	LOW	INTERMEDIATE	HIGH
Baked, canned	○		
Butter, dried and cooked	○		
Kidney, canned	○		
Lima, baby, frozen	○		
Mung, cooked	○		
Navy, dried and cooked	○		
Pinto, cooked	○		
Soy, canned	○		

Lentils

FOOD	LOW	INTERMEDIATE	HIGH
Green, dried and cooked	○		
Red, dried and cooked	○		

FOOD	LOW	INTERMEDIATE	HIGH
Peas			
Black-eyed	○		
Chickpeas/garbanzo beans, canned	○		
Split, yellow, cooked	○		

MEAL-REPLACEMENT PRODUCTS

FOOD	LOW	INTERMEDIATE	HIGH
Designer chocolate, sugar free, Worldwide Sport Nutrition low carbohydrate products	○		
L.E.A.N Fibergy bar, Harvest Oat, Usana	○		
L.E.A.N (Life long) Nutribar, Peanut Crunch, Usana	○		
L.E.A.N (Life long) Nutribar, Chocolate Crunch, Usana	○		

MIXED MEALS AND CONVENIENCE FOODS

FOOD	LOW	INTERMEDIATE	HIGH
Chicken nuggets, frozen, reheated	○		
Fish fillet, reduced fat, breaded	○		
Fish sticks	○		
Greek lentil stew with a bread roll, homemade	○		
Lean Cuisine, chicken with rice	○		
Pizza, Super Supreme, pan, Pizza Hut	○		
Pizza, Super Supreme, thin and crispy, Pizza Hut	○		
Pizza, Vegetarian Supreme, thin and crispy, Pizza Hut	○		
Spaghetti Bolognese	○		
Sushi, salmon	○		
Tortellini, cheese, Stouffer	○		
Tuna patty, reduced fat	○		
Cheese sandwich, white bread		◑	
Kugel		◑	
Macaroni and cheese, boxed, Kraft		◑	
Peanut-butter sandwich, white/whole-wheat bread		◑	
Pizza, cheese, Pillsbury		◑	

FOOD	LOW	INTERMEDIATE	HIGH
Spaghetti, gluten-free, canned in tomato sauce		◐	
Sushi, roasted sea algae, vinegar and rice		◐	
Taco shells, cornmeal-based, baked, El Paso		◐	
White bread and butter		◐	
Stir-fried vegetables with chicken and rice, homemade			●

NOODLES

FOOD	LOW	INTERMEDIATE	HIGH
Instant	○		
Mung bean, Lungkow beanthread	○		
Rice, fresh, cooked	○		
Rice, dried, cooked		◐	
Udon, plain, reheated 5 min		◐	

PASTA

FOOD	LOW	INTERMEDIATE	HIGH
Capellini	○		
Fettuccine, egg	○		
Gluten-free, cornstarch	○		
Linguine, thick, fresh, durum wheat, white	○		
Linguine, thin, fresh, durum wheat	○		
Macaroni, plain, cooked	○		
Ravioli	○		
Spaghetti, cooked 5 min	○		
Spaghetti, cooked 22 min	○		
Spaghetti, protein enriched, cooked 7 min	○		
Spaghetti, whole wheat	○		
Spirali, cooked, durum wheat	○		
Star pastina, cooked 5 min	○		
Tortellini	○		
Vermicelli	○		
Gnocchi		◐	

FOOD	LOW	INTERMEDIATE	HIGH
Rice vermicelli		◑	
Spaghetti, cooked 10 min, Barilla		◑	
Corn, gluten-free			●
Rice and corn, gluten-free			●
Rice, brown, cooked 16 min			●

PROTEIN FOODS

FOOD	LOW	INTERMEDIATE	HIGH
Beef	○		
Cheese	○		
Cold cuts	○		
Eggs	○		
Fish	○		
Lamb	○		
Pork	○		
Sausages	○		
Shellfish (shrimp, crab, lobster, etc.)	○		
Veal	○		

SNACK FOODS AND CANDY

Candy

FOOD	LOW	INTERMEDIATE	HIGH
Nougat	○		
Jelly beans			●
Life Savers			●
Skittles			●

Chips

FOOD	LOW	INTERMEDIATE	HIGH
Corn, plain, salted, Doritos	○		
Potato, plain, salted	○		

Chocolate bars

FOOD	LOW	INTERMEDIATE	HIGH
Milk, Cadbury's	○		

FOOD	LOW	INTERMEDIATE	HIGH
Milk, Dove, Mars	○		
Milk, Nestlé	○		
White, Milky Bar	○		
Mars Bar		◑	
Snickers Bar		◑	

Chocolate candy

M & M's, peanut	○		

Chocolate spread

Nutella, chocolate hazelnut spread	○		

Dried-fruit bars

Fruit Roll-Ups			●

Nuts

Cashews	○		
Peanuts	○		
Pecans	○		

Popcorn

Plain, microwaved			●

Pretzels

Plain, salted			●

Snack bars

Apple Cinnamon, ConAgra	○		
Peanut Butter & Choc-Chip	○		
Twix Cookie Bar, caramel	○		
Kudos Whole Grain Bars, chocolate chip		◑	

Sports bars

Ironman PR bar, chocolate	○		

FOOD	LOW	INTERMEDIATE	HIGH
PowerBar, chocolate		◐	

SOUPS

FOOD	LOW	INTERMEDIATE	HIGH
Lentil, canned	○		
Minestrone, canned, ready-to-serve	○		
Tomato, canned	○		
Black bean, canned		◐	
Green pea, canned		◐	
Split pea, canned		◐	

SPECIAL DIETARY PRODUCTS

FOOD	LOW	INTERMEDIATE	HIGH
Choice DM, vanilla, Mead Johnson	○		
Ensure, Abbott	○		
Ensure Plus, vanilla, Abbott	○		
Ensure Pudding, vanilla, Abbott	○		
Ensure bar, chocolate fudge brownie, Abbott	○		
Ensure, vanilla, Abbott	○		
Glucerna bar, lemon crunch, Abbott	○		
Glucerna SR shake, vanilla, Abbott	○		
Glucerna, vanilla, Abbott	○		
Resource Diabetic, vanilla, Novartis	○		
Resource Plus, chocolate, Novartis	○		
Ultracal with fiber, Mead Johnson	○		
Enercal Plus, Wyeth-Ayerst		◐	
Enrich Plus shake, vanilla, Ross		◐	

SUGARS

FOOD	LOW	INTERMEDIATE	HIGH
Blue Agave, Organic Agave Cactus Nectar, light, 90% fructose, Western Commerce	○		
Blue Agave, Organic Agave Cactus Nectar, light, 97% fructose, Western Commerce	○		
Fructose	○		

FOOD	LOW	INTERMEDIATE	HIGH
Lactose	○		
Honey		◑	
Sucrose		◑	
Glucose			●
Maltose			●

VEGETABLES

FOOD	LOW	INTERMEDIATE	HIGH
Artichokes	○		
Avocado	○		
Bok choy	○		
Broccoli	○		
Cabbage	○		
Carrots, peeled, cooked	○		
Cassava (yucca), cooked with salt	○		
Cauliflower	○		
Celery	○		
Corn, canned, no salt added	○		
Cucumber	○		
French beans (runner beans)	○		
Leafy greens	○		
Lettuce	○		
Peas, frozen, cooked	○		
Pepper	○		
Potato, sweet	○		
Squash	○		
Yam	○		
Beet		◑	
Corn, sweet, cooked		◑	
Potato, boiled/canned		◑	
Potato, new, canned		◑	
Taro		◑	

FOOD	LOW	INTERMEDIATE	HIGH
Broad beans			●
Parsnips			●
Potato, French fries, frozen and reheated			●
Potato, instant			●
Potato, mashed			●
Potato, microwaved			●
Potato, russet, baked			●
Pumpkin			●
Rutabaga			●

FOR MORE INFORMATION

To find a dietitian

The American Dietetic Association
120 South Riverside Plaza
Suite 2000
Chicago, IL 60606
Phone: 1-800-877-1600
www.eatright.org

To order Natural Ovens bread

Natural Ovens Bakery
PO Box 730
Manitowoc, WI 54221-0730
Phone: 1-800-772-0730
www.naturalovens.com

To order FIFTY50 Foods or find your nearest retailer:

FIFTY50 Foods

PO Box 89
Mendham, NJ 07945
Phone: 1-973-543-7006
www.fifty50.com

Primary Care Physicians

If you think you need help with a weight problem, it's always a good idea to see your primary care physician for an evaluation.

Community Support Groups

Many communities offer support groups targeting people who are trying to lose weight. Your primary care physician or local hospital may be able to direct you to a support group best suited to your needs.

Diabetes Organizations

Extra weight can often make a diabetic condition worse. For more information about living with and controlling your diabetes, contact the following:

The American Diabetes Association
1701 North Beauregard Street
Alexandria, VA 22311
Phone: 1-800-DIABETES (1-800-342-2383)
www.diabetes.org

Canadian Diabetes Association
National Office
15 Toronto Street, Suite 800
Toronto, ON M5C 2E3
Phone: 1-416-363-3373
1-800-BANTING (1-800-226-8464)
www.diabetes.ca

GLYCEMIC INDEX TESTING

*I*F YOU ARE a food manufacturer, you may be interested in having the glycemic index value of some of your products tested on a fee-for-service basis. For more information, contact:

Sydney University Glycaemic Index Research Service (SUGiRS)
Department of Biochemistry
University of Sydney
NSW 2006 Australia
Fax: (61) (2) 9351-6022
E-mail: j.brandmiller@staff.usyd.edu.au

ACKNOWLEDGMENTS

We would like to thank Linda Rao, M.Ed., for her editorial work on the American edition.

ABOUT THE AUTHORS

JENNIE BRAND-MILLER, PH.D., is Professor of Human Nutrition in the Human Nutrition Unit, School of Molecular and Microbial Biosciences at the University of Sydney, and President of the Nutrition Society of Australia. She has taught postgraduate students of nutrition and dietetics at the University of Sydney for over twenty-four years and currently leads a team of twelve research scientists, whose interests focus on all aspects of carbohydrate—diet and diabetes, the glycemic index of foods, insulin resistance, lactose intolerance, and oligosaccharides in infant nutrition. She has published sixteen books and 140 journal articles and is the coauthor of all books in the *Glucose Revolution* series.

■

KAYE FOSTER-POWELL, M. NUTR. & DIET., is an accredited practicing dietitian with extensive experience in diabetes management. She has conducted research into the glycemic index of foods and its practical applications over the last fifteen years. Currently she is a dietitian with Wentworth Area Diabetes Services in New South Wales and consults on all aspects of the glycemic index. She is the coauthor of all books in the *Glucose Revolution* series.

Also Available

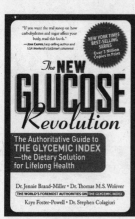

ISBN: 1-56924-506-1 • $15.95
ISBN-13: 978-1-56924-506-4

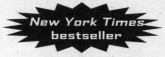

THE NEW GLUCOSE REVOLUTION

Written by the world's foremost authorities on the subject, whose findings are supported by hundreds of studies from Harvard University's School of Public Health and other leading research centers, *The New Glucose Revolution* shows how and why eating low-GI foods has major health benefits for everybody seeking to establish a way of eating for lifelong health.

THE LOW GI DIET REVOLUTION

The only science-based diet proven to help you lose up to 10 percent of your current weight and develop a lifetime of healthy eating habits that can protect you from illness and disease. *The Low GI Diet Revolution* shows you how to make low-GI food choices for every meal that will satisfy your hunger, increase your energy levels, and eliminate your desire to eat more than you should.

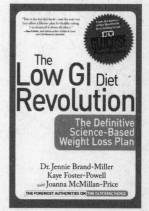

ISBN: 1-56924-413-8 • $15.95
ISBN-13: 978-1-56924-413-5

THE NEW GLUCOSE REVOLUTION LIFE PLAN

Both an introduction to the benefits of low-GI foods and an essential source for those already familiar with the concept, *The New Glucose Revolution Life Plan* presents the glycemic index within the context of today's full nutrition picture. With the glycemic index as its starting point, it gives readers clear guidelines for choosing the diet that is right for them. With the most authoritative, up-to-date and complete table of GI values published anywhere, *The New Glucose Revolution Life Plan* makes the glycemic index accessible and useful to more readers than ever before.

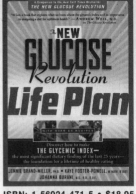

ISBN: 1-56924-471-5 • $18.95
ISBN-13: 978-1-56924-471-5

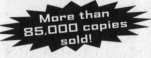

More than 85,000 copies sold!

THE NEW GLUCOSE REVOLUTION SHOPPER'S GUIDE TO GI VALUES 2006

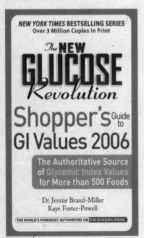

ISBN: 1-56924-329-8 • $6.95
ISBN-13: 978-1-56924-329-9

With GI values for hundreds of foods and beverages, this guide makes it easier than ever to ascertain a food's GI value. Included are two easy-to-read tables: an A to Z listing that specifies serving size, net carbohydrate per serving, and the glycemic load, and a handy, at-a-glance table sorted according to low, intermediate, and high-GI values.

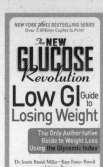

1-56924-336-7 • $6.95
ISBN-13: 978-1-56924-336-7

THE NEW GLUCOSE REVOLUTION LOW GI GUIDE TO LOSING WEIGHT

Learn how you can best use the glycemic index for effective weight loss. *The New Glucose Revolution Low GI Guide to Losing Weight* clearly describes the differences between carbohydrates and how low-GI foods can help you feel fuller longer, burn more body fat, and achieve and maintain a healthy weight and lifelong eating habits.

THE LOW GI DIET COOKBOOK

One hundred absolutely delicious, easy-to-make low-GI recipes—all of which feature low-GI carbohydrates—that will inspire you to adopt low-GI eating as *the* way to cook and eat—not only to keep your weight under control, but to improve and maintain your overall health and vitality, for life.

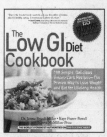

1-56924-359-X • $19.95
ISBN-13: 978-1-56924-359-X

THE NEW GLUCOSE REVOLUTION LOW GI EATING MADE EASY

A one-stop resource for those looking to switch to a healthy low-GI diet, this easy-to-follow guide features in-depth entries for the top 100 foods with the lowest GI values. Tips for making easy substitutions from high to low-GI foods and over 300 quick meal, snack, and treat suggestions are offered throughout.

1-56924-385-9 • $12.95
ISBN-13: 978-1-56924-385-5

Food manufacturers are showing increasing interest in having the GI values of their products measured. Some are already including the GI value of foods on food labels. As more and more research highlights the benefits of low-GI foods, consumers and dietitians are writing and telephoning food companies and diabetes organizations asking for GI data. This symbol has been registered in several countries, including the United States and Australia, to indicate that a food has been properly GI tested—in real people, not in a test tube—and also makes a positive contribution to nutrition. You can find out more about the program at www.gisymbol.com.au.

As consumers, you have a right to information about the nutrients and physiological effects of foods. You have a right to know the GI value of a food and to know it has been tested using appropriate standardized methodology.